12 Rounds

Bobby Whisnand

ISBN: 1523292709
ISBN-13: 978-1523292707

DEDICATION

Thanks Mom and Dad for all of my life lessons so greatly and lovingly taught to me which have guided me to exactly where I am today. I also want to thank all of my clients I have had over 25 years in the fitness business for listening to me run my mouth when I should have been counting reps. And, a big thank you to Dr. Harry Meyers, Dr. Lawrence Barzune, Dr. John Hollowell, Dr. Wayne "Buzz" Burkhead, Dr. John Racanelli, Dr. Louis Fox, and Dr. Victor Gonzalez, for trusting me with your patients through all of these years.

I have a goal I have not yet reached, and I'm just fine with that. My goal is to teach every person I see to live and feel as young as I do. So that you can always be able to do the things you love to do; regardless of how long you end up living. And I hope from the bottom of my big ole Texas heart, that in some way, I get to be a part of that with you.

Bring On The Fight!

CONTENTS

Introduction to 12 Rounds

Do you remember your first car? Man I sure do remember mine; it was a blue 1966 Chevrolet pickup that I thought was the best thing on four wheels. I took care of it like it was a Ferrari even though I only paid $600 for it. The thing is, it was mine, all mine, and I will never forget how powerful and exciting it felt to drive it to school, to my friend's houses, and out to the lake to fish. To others, it was a just another beat up old truck sounding like it was about to fall apart, but to me…it was a brand new truck that ran like a champ. It was my pride and joy and most importantly, it was the very first set of wheels I could call my own.

I think we all remember our first experiences of a lot of things in our lives like our first girlfriend or boyfriend, first day in high school, first job, that day we *finally* got our driver's license, and when we turned 21. But, there's one more thing for me that is probably not on many list of "first" out there… my first gym. That's right; the very first gym I belonged to was the one I built with my own two hands right inside our garage during the spring of my senior year in high school in 1986. I built a squat rack, a bench press, and an upright bench out of 2x6s and plywood. I also built a pulley system where I could do seated rows, lat pull downs, triceps push downs, cable curls, and other exercises. It wasn't much to look at, but just like that beat up truck, I thought it was awesome…and it was all mine.

That's exactly where it all started for me almost 30 years ago: Lifting bent and rusty bars loaded with as many of those grey concrete weights as I could handle in a hot unventilated garage that I called "My Gym". Where benches made from wood left imprints on my back that I thought would never go away, where cable and pulley configurations somehow held up, and where mismatched third hand weights laid in piles on the floor; my love and passion for exercise was born, and my life in fitness began.

Back then, my gym was a lot more to me than just a place to work out; it was a place where I felt great about myself, a place where I could make progress I could see, and a place where I always felt bigger and stronger than I really was; even if it was only for a short time. I learned a lot working out in that little gym and little did I know, the very things I learned way back then were the beginning of some of the most valuable things I have ever learned in all the years since, and I still use them today. I learned that improving yourself with exercise is a little different for all of us, and what works for one definitely isn't guaranteed to work for another. I learned it's not about how much you can lift but it's ALL about *how* you lift. I learned that true strength and fitness has absolutely nothing to do with how much you can bench press, squat, or curl, but more so about building a sound, strong, and balanced body by doing it right. And I learned that succeeding in improving your life with fitness goes way beyond exercising your body and eating well; it has just as much to do with training your mind to lead the way.

I took these very things I learned working out in that homemade gym and built a life and a career in fitness, not only helping myself achieve greater health, but helping thousands of others do the same. And now, it's your turn. In this book, I'm going to give you everything you need to take yourself to the next level of fitness, regardless of where you currently are. I'm going to walk you through 84 days of a program which has been tried, tested, and put through the ringer for many years that will prove to be the most effective, safe, individualized, and productive fitness program you will ever use. You're not only going to develop a strong, well balanced, and versatile body, you're going to become mentally stronger and self motivated to become healthier than you have ever been.

It's going to be a whole new experience for you because regardless of whether or not you currently exercise, I designed this program for you to go at it on your terms by doing it within your time and schedule, exercising at your own pace, making it convenient by having everything you need in one place, and making it fun and full of variety to keep you interested. You'll get to read some great stories about the experiences in my life, you'll get back in touch with the things you love to do, and at the end of 12 weeks, you'll have the means and method to do it again any time in your future, right there in the palm of your hands. So, are you wondering how this whole thing actually works? I'm going to show you right now.

Overview

You're about to start the most exciting and productive exercise program you have ever done or will ever do; 12 Rounds. You and I are going to do this together for the next 12 weeks (84 days) but before we start, I want you to read through this overview and "Keys to Victory" so you'll know what's coming your way and see exactly where we're headed. 12 Rounds is a completely holistic fitness program that is going to teach you how to exercise your body and mind in the best way possible, it's going to teach you how to eat well and manage your diet, you're going to restore your body's natural mobility, and you will learn to become self motivating in all parts of your life. You'll also learn how to manage stress, learn how to use visualization in exercise and self improvement, and do things you thought you would never be able to do again. Oh yeah, you'll get to hear a lot of stories from me as well; some funny, some motivating, and some emotional, but definitely ones you'll remember.

Each chapter of 12 Rounds will encompass one entire week where you will be led through every day whether it's an exercise day or not. Some days you'll exercise but other days you'll simply write a goal or two, log your food, take a few heart rates, or do something simple to help manage your stress. Don't worry; it's simple, fun, full of energy, and definitely life changing. What do you say we take a look at the actual sections you're going to see for each of the 12 rounds in this book? Let's do it.

It Happened Just Like This!

Each Round will begin with a story from my life experiences over the years, from my career, or from someone else's experiences they had in their life. These stories will set the tone for the entire Round and half way through the week, you'll get another story to read that will keep your interest high and motivate you to put forth your best effort. Whatever the story is, you'll like it, remember it, and you'll be able to use it at some point in your life to help you make a big change, or change just one little thing.

That One Thing

For three days a week I will ask you to do one simple task that will help improve your life. Some of the things I will be asking you to do are writing important things down, looking back over your workout or food journal, or to start writing a plan to remove a long overdue project or task that has been hanging over your head for a while. Either way, they are simple, easy to do, and will be an integral part of improving all parts of your life. You just have to make a plan to get it done and get it off your back and this is the perfect program to help you do just that.

Which Way You Headed?

This section will be your map to wherever it is you want to go. I'm going to teach you how to set attainable and realistic goals that will keep you on track during the next 12 weeks and beyond. You will be setting goals for exercising and eating well, but you will also set goals for your career, personal life, self image, finances, and many others. The best part is, we will write them as we go and we will never do more than three a week. Keep it simple right? It's one thing to set goals, but it's all together another thing to actually see yourself reaching those goals.

Seeing I to Eye

Your mind and your body are hard wired and what affects one will have considerable affects on the other. For this very reason, I have made visualization an integral part of my 12 Rounds program and by the time you reach the twelfth round, you'll be seeing I to eye with exactly what you want out of life. Throughout this program I will have you visualize many things about yourself like how you want to look, having unlimited energy, being happy, succeeding at your career, improving your social life or relationships, and definitely improving your health. Oh yea, using visualization before your workout is extremely powerful too; you'll definitely be on your game.

Pre Game

One thing I have found over my years in the fitness business and in my personal workouts is the fact that the better you are prepared *for* your workouts, the better and more productive your workouts will be. I'm going to give you exactly what you need to do before each of your workouts including both physical and mental things like when and what to eat, going over your workout before you do it, and getting your mind ready to knock it out of the park. When you're body and mind is optimally prepared to workout, everything goes to a whole new level and every one of your workouts will be a big win.

Your Workout

Oh yes! This is where things get very interesting. One thing for sure, we are all different in how our bodies and our minds respond to exercise but at the same time, there is one thing that all of us respond to both physically and mentally; variety! Keeping things interesting for both your body and mind is one of the most crucial parts of being successful in fitness. This is the very reason I have designed all of the workouts within 12 Rounds to holistically exercise your body in many different ways using many different methods to give you ultimate body balance and strength. With each round of this 12 round program, you will be given a list of things to apply to each week's workouts like a particular order of exercises, rest times between sets, and particular exercises you will do. The cool thing is… it will change for each of the 12 weeks and you will never do the same thing twice. Some things will be similar, but never exactly the same.

In addition, I'm going to give you the exact workouts I do, a shorter version in case you have very limited time, and instructions on how to apply each weeks specific variables and changes to the workout you're already doing if you so choose. Either way, your workouts are going to be exciting, new and a knockout every single week. To make things even better, I have every single workout written in your workout journal so all you have to do is fill in the blanks to keep track of everything you do. One more thing: You have to remember that what you do immediately *after* your workout is just as important as what you do before and during your workout. *Finishing* strong is the best way to make sure you start strong the next time.

Finishing Strong

One of the most neglected parts of fitness is not recuperating from your exercise session once you're done, but I'm definitely not going to let that happen to you. Once you're done with your workout, you're going to see a list of things you need to do to make sure you start recuperating your body and mind as fast as possible. You'll get post workout food recommendations, visualization techniques, and suggestions for completing your workout journal. It's great knowing you finished your workout strong and your body felt great doing it, but how did your heart do?

And The Heart Says…

Too many people judge their fitness level by how they look, how strong they are, and how far or fast they can run. Although these can be indicators of fitness, they are not the best ways to tell how fit you truly are. If you really want to know how effective your workouts are and how healthy you really are, you have to listen to your heart;

the most important muscle in your entire body. With this program, you're going to take heart rates all across each week including before, during, and after your workouts, and even on the days you do not work out. There's a heart rate table right before Day 1 and in the back of this book so be sure to use it often to make sure your heart is right where it should be. Your heart speaks volumes to you, you just have to listen to what it's telling you, especially when stress jumps on your back.

Upper Management

Stress is a part of life, but if you let it have its way, it will become a much bigger part of your life than you want it to be. Stress can be slow and sneaky or fast and hard hitting, but either way, it can and will keep you off track to getting what you want out of life. The key to managing stress is to not let it get the best of you so for this reason, I'm giving you little things each week of this program to help you not only manage stress, but to get rid of it as soon as you can. Managing stress has a lot to do with what you think but believe it or not, it also has a lot to do with what you eat.

Cleaning Your Plate

The absolute best thing you can do to improve your life with fitness is to first and foremost understand food and how it works in your body. Across each week I'm going to teach you about different types of food, how to time them within your diet to get the most out of them, and clear up major misconceptions about food that you're sure to run across. It's not only about what you eat; it's about when you eat it, the combinations of food you eat, and writing everything down so you can see exactly where you may be going wrong. That's exactly why I included a food journal just for you; don't get mad at me.

You Ate What??

You knew it was coming sooner or later, so here it is. I have built a food journal into every day of this program so you can keep track of EVERYTHING you are eating and drinking each day. I know, just what you wanted to hear right? Within this journal, you're going to keep track of total calories consumed, breakdown of proteins, carbohydrates, and fats, time of days that you're eating, and your water intake. The only way to keep things on track with your eating is to write everything down, but it will all pay off big time; I promise!

12 Rounds is the most comprehensive, fully encompassing, and detailed program you will find because it's designed to improve everything in your life on your terms. It's designed in a way that you can go at it according to your time and schedule, your abilities and goals, and your exercise preferences. It's full of variety and it's going to teach you how to exercise in the healthiest ways possible. It's going to teach you exactly what you should eat and why, and it's going to teach you how to train your brain to lead you to wherever it is you want to go. And the best thing about 12 Rounds; it's designed to help you whether you are an exercise fanatic, an occasional exerciser, or you have never exercised a day in your life.

12 Rounds will teach you to live life on your terms, succeed at things you never thought were possible, and get exactly what you want out of life. I'm in that place now and have been for a very long time, and I want the same for you. Are you ready to get going? It's almost time for you to snap it on tight and get going but before you do, I want to give you my ***"Keys To Victory"*** which will ensure you have amazing success with this program and most importantly, you'll come out a huge winner.

Everyone loves to win, and that's exactly what you're going to do with 12 Rounds. Up to this point, you've got a good idea of what this program is about with the different sections you're going to see throughout each week, but there are some very important things I want you to know before you start. These are my ***"Keys To Victory"*** and it's very important that you apply these to this program because it's these things that make 12 Rounds so unique and effective. Don't skip out on me; I'll know if you do.

Keep these things in your mind as you go through this program and don't hesitate to look back at this page at any time to get a good reminder.

Keys To Victory

1. Go at Your Own Pace - This is YOUR program; don't feel rushed to do more than you can do and try not to compare what you're doing to what others are doing in their workouts. Go at your own pace.

2. Listen to Your Heart - Make sure you take and record your heart rates when prompted and always refer to the heart rate chart in this book so you'll know the safe exercise ranges for your age. This program depends on you taking and recording heart rates so make sure you *don't skip a beat.*

3. Avoid Pain at All Cost - If you are doing a particular exercise with this program or any other program and you experience pain, stop doing the exercise all together, modify the exercise so no pain exist, or shorten the range of motion of the exercise. If pain persists, go see your doctor before continuing this or any exercise program.

4. Use Your Manual Everyday – This 12 Rounds program is designed for me to be with you every day for 12 weeks. Each day is different and is an integral part of this program so it's vital to your success that you have it with you every day. The best thing to do is to treat it just like your phone and take it to work, in your automobile, in your home, and on vacation when you go.

5. Always Fill Out Your Workout Logs – With as many changes as there are from week to week with this program, you absolutely have to keep an accurate log of each workout. This program builds from one week to the next and much of what you do depends on the outcomes from the previous weeks. The best thing to do is to fill it out after every set you do so you will be accurate and it won't take any time away from your workout. This is another crucial part of this program so make sure you make it a priority.

6. Be Honest and Diligent with Your Food Journal – I know this can be a little tedious but just like your workout log, your food journal is vital for this program to work for you. The benefits of a food log is you get to see exactly what and when you are eating, and it's the easiest and most effective way to see where you need to make changes. If you're not honest or if you leave some things off, the integrity of this program will be affected. Keep it honest and keep it clean.

7. Stay Hydrated – Make sure you have plenty of water before, during, and after you exercise. There will be suggestions for water intake on your workout days.

8. Follow This Program Exactly Like it is Designed – Like I stated earlier, this program builds upon itself from one day to the next and much of what you do from day to day depends on everything you have done on previous days. Believe it or not, the workouts in this program are not the biggest part of it; it's the other things like goal setting, planning, visualization, and stress management activities that are just as big and what make it so successful. You will have amazing success with 12 Rounds but to do so you have to take part in all 84 days. It will definitely be worth it, which you are soon to find out.

9. Give it Your Best Shot – Over the next 12 weeks, I'm going to take you through the most exciting and comprehensive program available today, but I need you to give me and this program your absolute best effort for it to be a great success in your life. Give this program everything you've got for the next 84 days and I promise to do the same for you.

10. Smile! You're going to do great things over the next 12 weeks.

There you have it: The keys to making my 12 Rounds the best program you have ever done. I'm very excited because I know what's about to happen for you. You're going to be amazed at a lot of things like how great you're going to feel, how much energy you're going to have, and how strong you're going to get. You're going to learn a lot of new things about exercise and nutrition, you'll learn how to set and meet new goals, and how to keep a positive outlook about life; even when tough times come around. There's one more thing I hope you get out of this program: I hope you have so much success that somewhere down the road, maybe even years after you complete this program, you think back and feel at least a little of what I felt 30 years ago working out in a hot garage in a little north Texas town in a rickety gym made from wood. Where the weights didn't match, the bars were bent and rusty, and the music was rock and roll. I loved everything about that little gym, but what I loved the most…it was where great and amazing things started to happen for me, and little did I know, it was just the beginning of a wonderful life.

Heart Rate

You'll be taking many heart rates throughout 12 Rounds, both on days you work out and on days where you don't. It's very important that you take all heart rates when prompted and record them as well because this will be one of your biggest indicators of how much healthier you're getting as you go through 12 Rounds.

Do you know how to take your heart rate? Just in case you don't here you go!

- Take your first two fingers on one hand and place them lightly just above your thumb where your wrist meets your hand; just like in the picture here.
- Next, slowly and lightly press down until you feel your pulse. This may take a few tries but you'll find it.
- Once you find your pulse, use your watch, phone, stopwatch, or second hand on a clock and count your pulse for six seconds.
- Take that number and simply add a zero. For example: If I took my pulse for six seconds and counted 8 beats, I would simply add a zero to 8 which would give me 80. Therefore, my pulse would be 80 beats a minute.

I have provided you with a heart rate chart both here and in the back of your workout log next to appendix A, so you can see what each heart rate means. You're going to be surprised by some of the heart rates you take within these 12 Rounds workouts because believe it or not; you're going to get aerobic activity from weight training alone. You'll see, and it's going to happen on your first workout.

I think it's a great idea to use a heart rate monitor every time you exercise so you can record much more than your heart rates. It's definitely not necessary but I do have a place for you to record heart rate monitor results if you choose to use one.

Age	Target HR Zone 50-85%	Average Maximum Heart Rate, 100%
20 years	100-170 beats per minute	200 beats per minute
30 years	95-162 beats per minute	190 beats per minute
35 years	93-157 beats per minute	185 beats per minute
40 years	90-153 beats per minute	180 beats per minute
45 years	88-149 beats per minute	175 beats per minute
50 years	85-145 beats per minute	170 beats per minute
55 years	83-140 beats per minute	165 beats per minute
60 years	80-136 beats per minute	160 beats per minute
65 years	78-132 beats per minute	155 beats per minute
70 years	75-128 beats per minute	150 beats per minute
75 years	73-123 beats per minute	145 beats per minute

Disclaimer

Make sure you have been released by your doctor to exercise. If you are currently involved in physical rehabilitation, finish your prescribed program and get a release from your physical therapist before starting this program.

If you have pain when you exercise, please stop and get checked out by your doctor before continuing.

If you feel light headed or become short of breath and cannot carry on a conversation, please stop exercising or greatly reduce the intensity of your exercise at once.

Please read

Not all of the exercises in this program are suitable for everyone and this or any exercise program may cause injury. To reduce the risk of injury, never force your body's range of motion or continue through pain. The methods, instruction, and suggested program are in no way a substitute for medical advice or counseling. The use of this product should only be conducted as stated in this program. The owners, producers, participants, distributors, and all affiliates of this program disclaim any and all liability or loss in connection with the exercises shown in this program, or the instruction and advice given herein.

In case you want to take and record your body measurements before you get started with 12 Rounds, I have the perfect place for you to do it. Remember, this is *YOUR* program and by no means do you have to measure anything. But if you want to, here you go!

Start of 12 Rounds Body Measurements

- **Date of measurements** - ___________________
- **Body weight** - _________ lbs
- **Body fat%** - ___________%
- **Shoulders** (measure across mid shoulder line) - _______
- **Chest** (measure across nipple line) - ________
- **Upper arm** (measure across mid bicep) - _______
- **Forearm** (measure across mid forearm between wrist and elbow) - _______
- **Waist** (measure right across belly button) - ________
- **Hips** (measure across mid buttocks) - ________
- **Upper thigh** (measure across mid upper thigh) - ________
- **Lower thigh** (measure across just above knee) - _______
- **Calf (measure across mid calf)** - _______

Round 1 – Light the Fire

Take a good look at yourself my friend because every single thing about you is about to change. The only things I ask of you are to stick to 12 Rounds exactly like I show you, go through every single day, and give me your best effort. Other than that, I'll do the rest. Are you ready to rock and roll? I'll see you at the top!

"The Heart of a Champion lives forever. It knows not of disadvantage, quit, or boasting. It lives within the soul and accepts the struggles of the fight like the air it breathes. It begins and ends every battle with the tenacity to fight to live another day. It knows not a cease in effort or passion to walk off the field of battle with a high head and a desire to do it over and over again; regardless of the outcome.

That's the Heart of a Champion." ***Bobby Whisnand***

Day 1

It Happened Just Like This!

I've had the pleasure of seeing thousands of people succeed at adding time and quality to their lives with fitness, and I want to tell you about one of them now. About 6 years ago, I received a call from the mother of a boy I trained while he was in high school. She said "Bobby, I really need your help with Justin. He's gained a lot of weight, he's depressed, and he never leaves the house except to go to his classes." She asked me to train with him again, and of course I agreed. Justin was 175 pounds when he graduated high school and four years later, he weighed 289 pounds.

I had a journal I designed that kept track of several things like workouts, goals, and food eaten. Justin and I started using it from the very first day and we would review it every week. After three months, Justin had lost 34 lbs, and you could see he was starting to get his confidence back. He did so well that I asked him to be in my upcoming exercise video, to which he happily agreed, and that very next year, he started working for me as a certified personal trainer. Today, he's my head trainer, my fitness coordinator, and he weighs 117 pounds less than he did when we started. Can you guess which program he still uses this very day? That's right: 12 Rounds. The very same program I use, and the same program I use for all of my clients because it works for everyone. And now…It's Your Turn!

That One Thing

For this first day of 12 Rounds, I want you to write down one thing you want to achieve the most with this program. Since 12 Rounds is designed to improve all parts of your life, it can be anything you want like losing weight, having a healthier heart, being more positive in the way you think, advancing in your career, improving your social life, or anything else you want. Go ahead and write that one thing and let's go make it come true.

1.____

Seeing I to Eye

My three biggest goals for you with this program are for you to feel amazing about who you are, for you to be proud of what you have accomplished, and for you to have more confidence than you've ever imagined. The key to achieving these three things starts with you being able to see it first, and that's exactly what we are going to do right now. At some point today, in a place that is quiet and without distractions, I want you to take just 2 minutes to relax and visualize yourself doing something you love to do. It can be going to a favorite vacation spot, something recreational, being with your favorite person, making money, getting an award, or anything else that's positive and fun for you. After you figure it out, write a brief description of it here. Make it a good one!

Pre Game

You have a workout coming up today and to make it the best possible, do these things before you go:

- ➔ Schedule your workouts just like a work appointment.
- ➔ Make sure you eat 1.5-2 hours before you exercise.
- ➔ Review your workout so you know what to expect.
- ➔ Drink plenty of water before you workout.
- ➔ If you are taking supplements, make sure you have them with you and take them at the right times.
- ➔ Take a few minutes before your workout and clear your mind.

Every workout you do will be different in many ways and will have its own personality; you'll see what I mean. At the beginning of every workout, I'm going to give you a list of specific things you will apply to that particular day's workout. At this point, you'll have three choices: You can apply these specific variables to the workout you're already doing, you can do the exact workout I'm giving you for that day, or you can do an abbreviation of this same workout if you have time constraints.

One point I want to make about your workouts is this: If you are just starting to work out or you have not worked out in the last month or longer, please use the abbreviated workout that's in **bold** for 3-4 weeks so you don't overdo anything. Do we have a deal? Good!

Lastly, I have written out every single workout you'll be doing in the appendix in the back of your workout journal, and the workouts you'll see there are my actual workouts with the exact weights and repetitions that I do. The reason I did this is for you to be able to take a look at how the amounts of weights change from one workout to the next because each workout is vastly different. If you will simply figure the percentage of difference from one week to the next, you'll be able to predict very closely what weights you'll be using for your own workouts.

One more very important thing about your workouts: The amount of time you rest between your sets varies from one workout to the next and it's crucial for the success of this program that you don't change any of the rest times. If you are limited on time, just do the workout in **bold,** but no matter what, keep the rest times between sets exactly like I have them.

I have included web links in your workout log so that you can see exactly how each of the warmups, exercises, and stretches should be performed. For the best results, I suggest that you look over the exercise log well in advance of your workouts, so that you know exactly what you will be doing before you start your workout program.

Your Workout - See your workout log for today's workout.

And the Heart Says…

I know you took a few heart rates during your workout today, but there are other times you need to take it as well. Tonight when you are lying in bed and before you go to sleep, take one more heart rate and write it down here.

Pre Sleep HR - ______ Time taken - _______

Cleaning Your Plate

There are many misconceptions about food, millions of opinions on what we should and shouldn't eat, and diet fads popping up every day. To avoid getting confused, the best thing you can do for yourself in terms of eating healthy is to learn about the different types of food and how they interact with your body. Throughout this book, I'll be giving you many of those things in this section but I'll also be giving you resources where you can find great information on nutrition. Today, we are going to start with the absolute best thing you can do to start eating healthier, and that's journaling your food. Make sure you have your food journal with you everyday so you can immediately write down your food and drink after every meal. Be honest now!

For the first few days, I only want you to write down what you ate and the time you ate it. You don't have to count calories or anything else at this point. As we go along, I'll ask you to add things like the amount of proteins, carbohydrates and fats as well as total calories, but for now, I just want you to get in the habit of journaling your food. Do we have a deal? Good!

You Ate What?

As you can see, there are five meals listed here. This doesn't mean you have to eat all five meals, it's just there in case you already do. But, as you can probably tell, 4-5 meals a day is what I will eventually ask you to eat. Everybody likes to eat, right?

Food Journal

Time of meal 1 - _________

Food eaten- ________________________________

____

Drink - ________________________________

Time of meal 2 - _________

Food eaten- ________________________________

____

Drink - ________________________________

Time of meal 3 - _________

Food eaten- ________________________________

____

Drink - ________________________________

Time of meal 4 - _________

Food eaten- ________________________________

____

Drink - ________________________________

Time of meal 5 - _________

Food eaten - ____

Drink - ________________________________

Congratulations on completing Day 1 of Round 1; I can't wait for you to see what's in store for Day 2. Tomorrow, I'm going to get you started on managing that "S" word but for now, eat some good clean food, get plenty of sleep, and I'll be right here waiting for you tomorrow. Great Job!

Round 1, Day 2

Good Morning! How did you sleep last night? I hope well, because today is a brand new day full of new things for you. Get your coffee, let the dog out, get ready for work, and let's get started.

Which Way You Headed?

Let's get this day started great by setting your first goal for this program. Today I want you to set one long term goal that you want to reach by the end of 12 Rounds (12 weeks), but I want this first goal to be about something other than fitness or your career. For example: it could be a goal on improving your finances, social life, relationship, or personal growth. After you've thought about it for a bit, write it down here.

My first long term (12 week) goal about something other than my fitness or my career is...

Seeing I to Eye

Believe me when I tell you this: One of the most productive ways to improve things about your life is to get good at visualizing. I know it's not easy at first but once you get good at it, you'll want to do it more. Today, I want you to find a quiet place without distractions where it's just you; leave that phone behind too. Once you're there, close your eyes, relax, take a few deep breaths, and visualize yourself exactly as you are at that very moment. Visualize your clothes (if you're wearing any... or not), your hair, your shoes, and put a smile on your face while you're at it. Do this for 2 minutes and that's it. See, I told you it would be easy. Now, let's talk about that stress in your life.

Upper Management

Stress is a natural part of life and it comes in three forms; the good, the bad, and the ugly. The key is to not let one turn into the other by managing it and getting rid of it as soon as you can. Over the course of 12 Rounds, I'm going to show you how to get rid of it as quick as you can so you don't pull all of your hair out, or someone else's. You can start right now by taking a deep breath, let it out slowly, think of something positive, and *relaxxxxxx*. Are you ready for your workout today? Let's see.

Pre Game

Always eat 1.5-2.5 hours before your workout, drink plenty of water before you workout, and keep positive thoughts in that head of yours. Don't forget your workout journal.

Your Workout - See your workout log for today's workout.

Cleaning Your Plate

"Exercise is a lot like food; it's great in its natural state, but it's how we use it that can make it bad."

Bobby Whisnand

There are three main things that can make food bad; how it's grown, how it's cooked, and how it's eaten. Try to eat organic and unprocessed foods as much as you can, cook your food in healthy ways, and control and measure how much you are eating.

You Ate What?

Just like for Day 1, just simply write down what you eat and drink and the times you consumed them. No cheating either.

Food Journal

Time of meal 1 - _________

Food eaten- ________________________________

____

Drink - ________________________________

Time of meal 2 - _________

Food eaten- ________________________________

____

Drink - ________________________________

Time of meal 3 - _________

Food eaten- ________________________________

____

Drink - ________________________________

Time of meal 4 - _________

Food eaten- ________________________________

____

Drink - ________________________________

Time of meal 5 - _________

Food eaten - ____

Drink - ________________________________

And The Heart Says…

Tonight after you eat and are sitting down relaxing, take a heart rate and write it down here:

After dinner HR-________ **Time taken -** _______

That's the completion of Day 2 my friend; now get some sleep because tomorrow's workout is going to be a tough one. It's LEG DAY!!

Round 1 – Day 3

Are you ready to get this Day 3 going? I am, and it's one of my favorite days because it's LEG DAY! Let's get it going.

That One Thing

To start this day off, I want you to write down one thing you think will help you have success with this program. I'm talking about things like… you enjoy working out, your determination, your support from others, you're eager to change your life, or you're good at working out, etc.

One thing that will help me have success with this program is…

____

Seeing I to Eye

Go to that secluded place you have and visualize yourself doing something fun, but this time add sounds, colors, voices, and other things you might feel if you were really there. Try it; it's easier than you think. Remember, before you start your visualization, always close your eyes, take a few deep breaths, and clear your mind.

Pre Game

Today is leg day and this is the workout that is a catalyst to growth and strength for all other muscles so make it a good one. Don't forget to stay hydrated before, during, and after your workout, eat 1.5-2.5 hours before you workout, and clear your mind of that stress.

Your Workout – See your workout log for today's workout.

And the Heart Says…

While you're in bed tonight but before you go to sleep, take one more heart rate and record it here.

Pre sleep HR - ______ Time taken - __________

Cleaning Your Plate

Do you know the difference between simple and complex carbohydrates (sugars)? When you hear the word "sugar" floating around in conversations about diets, most people are referring to the simple sugars which are in sweet foods and sweeteners. Examples of these are syrups, table sugar, desserts, sodas, candy, and sweet drinks. These types of simple refined and processed sugars should be avoided because they are cheap nutrition and will leave you tired and lethargic because they lack complete nutrition. Another simple sugar is that which is found in fruits but the difference is… these sugars are natural unless they have been processed like in many fruit juices and fruit drinks. Simple sugars are simple because they are absorbed in your blood stream very quickly within minutes after consuming them. Natural simple sugars are also very short lived as energy but if you eat them at the right times and they are not processed, they provide quick clean energy. Now, let's talk about the "other sugar".

Complex carbohydrates are sugars too, the difference is, they are absorbed much more slowly into your blood stream and they are a much longer lasting source of energy. Examples of complex carbs are grains, bread, pasta, rice, potatoes, beans, and legumes. These are the foods which provide sustained energy but they are also the ones where you have to limit how much you eat, especially if you are trying to lose weight. We will talk more about this in a few days.

Here is a great resource if you want to learn about the Glycemic Index which shows you how slow or fast different foods are absorbed into your blood stream.

http://www.diabetes.org/food-and-fitness/food/what-can-i-eat/understanding-carbohydrates/glycemic-index-and-diabetes.html

You Ate What?

Okay, the moment of truth. Make sure you write down EVERYTHING you eat and drink. Just think, the worse it is now, the greater your improvement will be later. And yes, that coffee you drink and everything you put in it counts so don't forget about writing it down too.

Food Journal

Time of meal 1 - ________

Food eaten- ______________________________

____

Drink - ______________________________

Time of meal 2 - ________

Food eaten- ______________________________

____

Drink - ______________________________

Time of meal 3 - ________

Food eaten- ______________________________

____

Drink - ______________________________

Time of meal 4 - ________

Food eaten- ______________________________

____

Drink - ______________________________

Time of meal 5 - ________

Food eaten - ____

Drink - ______________________________

You have reached the end of Day 3; what a day for you! It was leg day and you spent a lot of energy during your workout so make sure you get good clean food to eat for the remainder of your day, fill out that food journal, get something positive in your head, and go dream of something good. See you tomorrow!

Round 1, Day 4

There you are! How did you sleep last night? Today is Day 4, and the biggest difference is...NO WORKOUT TODAY! That's right, there are a few other things I want you to do but in terms of working out, there will be none of that today. You need days off for your body to recuperate and the best time to take it easy is the day after leg day. Let's go get this Day 4; you ready?

"To get the most out of life, you'll have to go through many times where it gets the most out of you"

Bobby Whisnand

It Happened Just Like This!

I'm definitely not one to be intimidated, but there was one day in my life where I was, and I'll never forget it. It was 1994 and I was at the Cooper Aerobics Institute in Dallas about to start my very first personal trainer certification and all I heard everyone talking about was how many certifications they had and how many years they had been personal training. They were also talking about how the Cooper Clinic certification was the most prestigious at that time and one of the most comprehensive. I thought, "Oh heck, I might be over my head. Maybe I should take a few other certifications before this one." But that feeling didn't last long because after a few exercise demonstrations and listening to others talk about how they trained their clients, I knew I was in the right place. And better yet, I knew I was better prepared to train people than anyone else there.

I guess you could say the most important and effective things I have learned about fitness came from seven years of attending the school of hard knocks. I tried what everyone else told me to do in exercise including countless different programs but none of it worked for me. I had to go through days, months, and years trying many different things hoping something would turn out right for me and little by little, I pieced it all together. Do you want to know the most valuable thing I learned over those seven years? I'll give you a hint; it has nothing to do with exercise and eating right. The most valuable thing I learned was how to stay tough and fight for a better life, and I'm going to teach you to do the same.

Which Way You Headed?

On Day 2, you wrote down one long term goal about something other than fitness. Today, write one long term goal (12 weeks) about your fitness like weight loss/gain, increasing energy, exercising for a certain amount of time per week, attaining a certain body measurement like body fat %, or anything else about fitness.

My first long term fitness goal is...

Seeing I to Eye

When you're in a quiet place without distractions, take 2 minutes and visualize yourself how you want to look physically. You can start by visualizing just one part of your body like your arms or legs or you can shoot for your entire body. I know this can be challenging but it's important for you to do it. This takes practice and time so don't be concerned if you have a hard time doing it. You'll have plenty of opportunity over the next 12 weeks to get good at it.

NO WORKOUT TODAY! – One of the biggest mistakes made in fitness is working out way too much. You have to give your body rest and the day after leg day is the perfect day to do just that. Take it easy today and enjoy your day off. Now if we could only get your boss to think the same way. Do you want me to call them?

Upper Management

One of the best ways to avoid stress is to plan ahead for things so they go smoothly. One thing I do every night before I go to bed is get everything ready for the next day so I don't have to rush the next morning. I absolutely don't like to get up early so if I can sleep longer by getting things ready the night before, I'm all in on that one. Think of something you can start doing in terms of planning ahead to avoid getting in a stressful situation and write it down here. Make this one something simple.

To avoid getting stressed, I'm going to plan ahead by…

And the Heart Says…

When you're sitting at your desk sometime this morning or just sitting around, take a heart rate and write it here –

Morning resting HR______ Time taken - ________

Cleaning Your Plate

Earlier this week I talked to you about the difference in simple and complex carbohydrates (sugars), and now I want to show you how eating too many carbohydrates at one time or across the course of a day can cause you to gain unwanted body fat. It's very simply a matter of having too much nutrition in your body at once. Your body will break down those carbohydrates (especially the complex ones) and store them in one of two places; in your blood as glucose and in your muscles as glycogen (stored energy). When your body senses you have enough glucose and glycogen stored up, the next thing to do is to store the excess nutrition as body fat. This is exactly why I tell anyone who is trying to drop body fat to greatly reduce the amount of complex carbohydrates they eat later in the day and to also cut out most simple carbohydrates with the exception of fruit.

On the other hand, if you are trying to gain weight, adding complex carbohydrates to each meal is a great way to do it. If gaining weight is your goal, slowly add complex carbohydrates into your diet in small increments across the day and don't forget to record these additions to your diet in your food journal.

You Ate What?

Okay now, this is the last day where you're only going to write down what and when you ate and drank something. Starting tomorrow, we're going to add total calories to the list. You might just be surprised at what you find.

Food Journal

Time of meal 1 - _________

Food eaten- ________________________________

____

Drink - ________________________________

Time of meal 2 - _________

Food eaten- ________________________________

____

Drink - ________________________________

Time of meal 3 - ________

Food eaten- ______________________________

____

Drink - ______________________________

Time of meal 4 - ________

Food eaten- ______________________________

____

Drink - ______________________________

Time of meal 5 - ________

Food eaten - ____

Drink - ______________________________

There you go; Day 4 is in the books! How are you feeling about things? Are you learning anything? I'm sure you are but there are a lot more things you're going to learn in the days to come. Okay, I'll shut up so you can go relax, eat some good food, and get some sleep. Tomorrow is back and bicep day, so you get to show off your guns. See you tomorrow!

Round 1, Day 5

There's always one good thing you can count on about Day 5 before the day even gets going for you; IT's FRIDAY! That's right, the end of the work week for some people and the start of unwinding, going out, and maybe even a little partying. It's all good: Just be safe, and don't forget to invite me. But you do have a workout today and tomorrow so don't forget to work those in.

That One Thing

To start the day off, think of one person with whom you can share your goals and progresses throughout 12 Rounds. Once you know who it is, write their name down here:

____

Seeing I to Eye

At some point today, take 3 minutes in that quiet place you go to and visualize working out. Picture yourself doing an exercise you like to do and see yourself being strong, in control, and getting a great pump. Be as specific as you can by seeing your clothes, hearing the sounds of the gym, and of course one of your favorite songs playing. Now go for it!

Pre Game

Make sure you're fully ready for your workout today; you know what to do.

Your Workout – See your workout log for today's workout.

And the Heart Says…

When you get home, sit down, rest for about a minute, take a heart rate, and write it down here.

Evening resting HR ______ Time taken - _______

Cleaning Your Plate

One of the most debated and misunderstood topics in nutrition today is the subject of fats. It's also an area where many people make big mistakes in their diets because they simply have been misinformed. Instead of giving you a ton of information on different types of fats found in foods and which ones are good and bad for you, I'm going to give you a great resource where you can start learning about fats. This link is from the Mayo Clinic and it will get you started with all the information you need. We will cover the specifics on fats very soon; don't worry.

http://www.mayoclinic.org/healthy-lifestyle/nutrition-and-healthy-eating/in-depth/fat/art-20045550

You Ate What?

There's one small addition to your food journal today. I want you to start writing the total calories for everything you eat and drink. Yep, the truth is upon you.

Food Journal

Time of meal 1 - _________

Food eaten- ________________________________

____

Drink - ________________________________

Total Calories - _________

Time of meal 2 - _________

Food eaten- ________________________________

____

Drink - ________________________________

Total Calories - _________

Time of meal 3 - _________

Food eaten- ________________________________

____

Drink - ________________________________

Total Calories - _________

Time of meal 4 - _________

Food eaten- ________________________________

____

Drink - ________________________________

Total Calories - _________

Time of meal 5 - _________

Food eaten - ____

Drink - ________________________________

Total calories - _________

Guess what? That's right; it's Friday and you have almost finished Round 1. Tomorrow you have a special workout that combines cardiovascular and core exercises and you're going to need your energy and endurance for this one. Go clear that head of yours, relax, visualize some positive things in your life, and I'll be waiting for you tomorrow for Day 6! Sleep tight.

Round 1 - Day 6

Hey Champ, It's great to see you today! Are you ready to rock and roll? I am because you're going to love today's workout. But before we get to it, there are a few things I want you to do. You ready?

Which Way You Headed?

So far this week you have written two goals; one about something other than fitness and one about fitness. Today, I want you to write one long term (12 week) goal about your career. It can be something like getting a promotion, getting noticed by your boss, taking on a big project, or anything else you want. Just make sure it's about your career. Okay, once you know what it is, write it down here:

My first long term (12 week) goal about my career is -

Upper Management

On Day 4, we talked about planning ahead to avoid stress. The other part of planning ahead is having alternate plans. Think about driving in a big city: If you know ahead of time there is a major traffic jam on your normal route to where you're going, you can adjust and take an alternate route to avoid the whole thing. But if you didn't know another route, you're going to be stuck in a mess and frustrated to no end; I know I would be. This same thing happens in all parts of our lives and not just on the freeways. Life happens, and it changes on a dime so plan ahead, have alternate plans, and have smooth sailing my friend. No Whammies!!

Seeing I to Eye

Before you workout today, take three minutes and visualize yourself running, biking, boxing, swimming, or doing any other endurance event and having extremely high energy where you feel you'll never run out. As a bonus, try visualizing today as you workout; it's harder to do because you're tired but it's amazingly effective. Don't forget to add all the good stuff like sounds, other people, and music.

Pre Game

Here's a brief reminder of the things you need to do before your workout to make it the best possible:

- Schedule your workouts just like a work appointment.
- Make sure you eat 1.5-2 hours before you exercise.
- Review your workout so you know what to expect.
- Drink plenty of water before you workout.
- If you are taking supplements, make sure you have them with you and take them at the right times.

- Take a few minutes before you workout and clear your mind.

Your Workout – See your workout log for today's workout.

And the Heart Says…

You took a lot of heart rates today but that's a good thing. I want you to take one more so we can see how your heart is recovering from that awesome workout today. At some point this evening when you are relaxed, take another heart rate and record it here.

Post workout HR ______ Time taken - _______

Cleaning Your Plate

Proteins are the building blocks of the body, essential for hormone production, and absolutely necessary for lean muscle growth and sustainability. I will be discussing proteins and their importance at different times over the course of 12 Rounds but to get you started, I'm going to give you a link about proteins where you can learn why they are so important for your body and exactly how your body uses them. Check out this link to WebMD for some great information of proteins. I'll be quizzing you later so be sure you check it out.

http://www.webmd.com/men/features/benefits-protein

You Ate What?

Are you getting good at writing your food and drink down? I know it can be tedious but it's a very big key to your success with this program so make it a part of your day. Don't forget those total calories today.

Food Journal

Time of meal 1 - _________	**Time of meal 2 - _________**
Food eaten- ________________________________	**Food eaten- ________________________________**
________________________________	________________________________
Drink - ________________________________	**Drink - ________________________________**
Total Calories - _________	**Total Calories - _________**
Time of meal 3 - _________	**Time of meal 4 - _________**
Food eaten- ________________________________	**Food eaten- ________________________________**
________________________________	________________________________
Drink - ________________________________	**Drink - ________________________________**
Total Calories - _________	**Total Calories - _________**

Time of meal 5 - ________

Food eaten - ____

Drink - ________________________________

Total calories - ________

You've almost completed your first round of my 12 Rounds program; how are you feeling about the whole thing at this point? From where I'm sitting, you're doing awesome and the best news is, it will only get better from here on out. Rest up, eat some good food, keep it positive, and I'll see you tomorrow for Day 7. Great Job!

Round 1 - Day 7

Are you awake yet? It's okay, today is the perfect day to take it easy because I'm going to give you a break from everything. I'll go ahead and give you a place to log a heart rate and a place to keep your food journal but you absolutely don't have to do anything except take it easy and have some fun. Tomorrow is the start of Round 2; a brand new round full of new workouts, new information about food, pushing toward reaching those goals, and new ways to manage that stress.

Now go have some fun and if it's something really fun, kind of crazy, and "out there", call me; I don't want to miss out.

Day 7 HR _____ **Time taken -** ______

You Ate What???

You do not have to fill this out today but if you want to, here it is; go for it!

Food Journal

Time of meal 1 - ________

Food eaten- ____________________________

____

Drink - ______________________________

Total Calories - ________

Time of meal 2 - ________

Food eaten- _______________________________

____

Drink - ______________________________

Total Calories - ________

Time of meal 3 - ________

Food eaten- ________________________________

____

Drink - __________________________________

Total Calories - ________

Time of meal 4 - ________

Food eaten- __________________________________

____

Drink - _________________________________

Total Calories - ________

Time of meal 5 - ________

Food eaten - ____

____

Drink - __________________________________

Total calories - ________

Round 2 – The Confidence Builder

Here we are; the start of a whole new round which you're going to love! Just like I said in the introduction of this book, every round is different and all 12 Rounds build upon each other as we go. Don't forget to take a look at the appendix in the back of your workout journal so you can get an idea of how much weight you're going to need for this week's workouts and always take those heart rates. Okay, enough of that; bring on Round 2!

"Always believe you can do great things in your life with what you currently have, and then go do it. There are many less fortunate people in this world doing a lot more with a lot less."

Bobby Whisnand

Day 1

It Happened Just Like This!

You know how there are certain people you run across in your life that you never forget? I've known several in my life but there's one that is a big part of who I am today. It was my very first year of personal training and a man came into the gym one morning and he asked, "Where are your elevators? I have a friend who wants to look at the gym but he's in a wheelchair and we can't get down those stairs." I told him the stairs were the only way down here and that I wished I could help out more. He thanked me and started walking out but before he got to the door, I told him I might have an idea. We walked upstairs and when we opened the door, there sat a man in his wheelchair, smiling as he stuck his hand out to meet me and he said, "I'm Gerald, how in the heck do we get to the gym downstairs?" That was all I needed to hear. We carried Gerald up and down two flights of stairs for three days a week and it was definitely a workout for all three of us, but it was damn well worth it.

The workouts were a challenge as well because we did all exercises out of his wheelchair, and I'll never forget; we used rope to secure Gerald to the bench press and different exercise machines to keep him from falling out. Every workout with Gerald was a challenge, but everything he taught me by the way he lived was more than worth it. I would ask him if he was ready for more weight and his response was always the same, "If you're waiting on me, you're backing up." Every workout we did together inspired me to no end, but one day he told something that changed me forever. He said, "Bobby, coming down here to workout with you is the best part of my life. Even if it's just for an hour, I forget all about being in that wheelchair and I feel there's nothing I can't do. Thanks for being here buddy."

It's very easy to take things for granted in our lives, complain about little insignificant things, and feel dejected when things don't turn out the way we want. The next time you find yourself in a situation like this, think of Gerald and the millions of people less fortunate than you, let yourself be humbled, and go make the most of what you have.

That One Thing

Last week you wrote down that one thing you wanted to achieve the most with this program. Write it down again here and also write down one thing you think could keep you from achieving it. Obstacles are everywhere; see yours before it sees you.

The one thing I want to achieve the most with this program is…

The one thing that could keep me from achieving it is ...

___

Seeing I to Eye

Go to that quiet place and for 3 minutes visualize something from your past that was a lot of fun. Once you can see yourself doing it, add sounds, color, voices, the wind, sun, and other things. If you have a favorite song, add it too.

Write down what you visualized here:

___

Pre Game

Are you ready for your workout? Make sure you eat some good food, drink plenty of water, and get your mind ready. Enjoy your workout, record all of your weights used in your journal, and take those heart rates.

Your Workout – See your workout log for today's workout

Please read before doing today's workout

Before you get to today's workout, I want to explain a few things because this week's workouts are vastly different than last weeks. Every workout this week involves **unilateral movements** which basically mean doing exercises with one arm or one leg at a time. Here's an example of doing an exercise unilaterally:

Dumbbell Shoulder Press – Let's say the first set you do is for 10 reps, you would do 10 repetitions with one arm, stop, and then do 10 reps with the other arm. That would complete the first set. You would repeat this for all sets to be done. However, there is one very important thing to remember with unilateral exercises and it has to do with your rest time between your sets. As soon as you complete the reps with the first arm, you would start your timer and continue on to the other arm. This is where you have to be very aware of your timer because you're timing the rest between each arm independently. By the time you get done with the second arm, the timer will tell you that you are almost ready to start with the first arm again.

The only exception to this is with the last set where you won't start the timer until you are done with the second arm. Then, for your last set, you'll start with the arm with which you finished on the first sets. Another thing I want you to take note of is that, at the beginning of each unilateral workout, I will tell you which arm or leg with which to start each exercise. This is important because the next time you do unilateral exercises you will start with the opposite side with which you started last time. This will balance everything out because you don't want to start with the same side for every workout using a unilateral method. To see a video of what unilateral exercises look like, use this link: **http://tinyurl.com/unilateralexercises**

Lastly, before you workout today, look at the Appendix in the back of your workout log where you can see the exact weights I used for the same exact workouts you're doing. What I want you to see is how the weights change when you do the exercises unilaterally vs. normal. If you will simply do the math and look at the differences in percentages of weights used when doing them unilaterally, you'll have a very good idea of the amount of weight you'll need for all exercises this week or any week for that matter. Take a look before you work out today but don't be making fun of me for using so little weight. I'm serious!

And the Heart Says…

I know you took a few heart rates before and after your workout today, but there are other times you need to take it as well. Tonight when you are lying in bed and before you go to sleep, take one more heart rate and write it down here.

Pre Sleep HR - ______ Time taken - ________

Cleaning Your Plate

At some point today, take a look at the label of one of the foods you eat and read through the ingredients. How many things do you see that you don't know what they are? Many foods are not what they seem because of processing which strips much of the nutrition from the food and adds bad things for you like preservatives and other chemicals. When looking for whole foods to eat, the ingredients should be a very short list of things and should only contain whole unprocessed foods.

You Ate What?

Starting today, start recording how many grams of carbohydrates you are getting with each meal. I'm talking about total carbs at this point; you don't have to differentiate between simple, complex, and fiber. Not yet that is! Don't forget those total calories as well.

Food Journal

Time of meal 1 - _________

Food eaten- ________________________________

____

Drink - ____________________________________

Total Carb Grams -_____ Total Calories - _____

Time of meal 2 - _________

Food eaten- ___________________________________

____

Drink - ______________________________________

Total Carb grams - _____ Total Calories - _______

Time of meal 3 - _________

Food eaten- ________________________________

____

Drink - ____________________________________

Total Carb Grams -_____ Total Calories - _____

Time of meal 4 - _________

Food eaten- ___________________________________

____

Drink - ______________________________________

Total Carb grams - ______ Total Calories - _______

Time of meal 5 - ________

Food eaten - ____

Drink - ____________________________________

Total Carb Grams -______ **Total Calories -** _______

And just like that, Day 1 of Round 2 is complete. What did you think about that workout today? It's a lot different than what you did on Round 1 right? This is what makes 12 Rounds so good; you're always giving your body and mind something different every day. Make sure you eat some good food, rest that body and mind with a good eight hours of sleep, think about something good, and I'll see you tomorrow for Day 2.

Round 2 - Day 2

Good morning! How's that body feel today? Let's get you going because today is your core and cardio day so let's get to it. Oh yea, don't be skipping breakfast either; I'll know if you do.

Which Way You Headed?

Last week you wrote down one long term goal about something other than fitness. Today, write that goal again and this time, write one short term goal (something you can realistically reach in two weeks) that will help you reach that long term goal

My first long term (12 week) goal for something other than fitness is...

____

My first short term (2 week) goal to help me reach this long term goal is...

____

Seeing I to Eye

Find that quiet place and for 3 minutes visualize yourself doing one thing at which you have little confidence in doing. Maybe it's public speaking, playing an instrument, singing, starting a conversation with the opposite sex, leading a study group or project, etc.

Write down what you visualize here:

____

Upper Management

One of the quickest ways stress becomes bad is when the things you need to do start to pile up on you. You know exactly what I mean don't you? We all do, so for that reason, I want you to write a list (short or long) of things that you need to get done which you have been putting off for some time now. You can add to this list as you go. I know; great news huh?

These are the things I need to get done to lighten my load:

1. ______________________ 7. ______________________

2. ______________________ 8. ______________________

3. ______________________ 9. ______________________

4. ______________________ 10. ______________________

5. ______________________ 11. ______________________

6. ______________________ 12. ______________________

Pre Game

How much water have you drunk today? Are you timing your meals so that you've eaten 1.5-2.5 hours before your workout? Make it a priority to do these things before all of your workouts.

Your Workout – See your workout log for today's workout

Cleaning Your Plate

Find a food label and review the nutrition breakdown. Pay close attention to how the carbohydrates are broken down into three main groups: total carbs, fiber, and sugars. To determine how many of the total carbs are complex, simply subtract the sugars and fiber from the "total carbs" and that number will give you the number of complex carbs per serving in that particular food. Start thinking about this today when you journal your food because it's coming soon.

You Ate What???

This food journal is starting to really take shape. Don't forget to write those total carbohydrates for each of your meals. Are you remembering to write down those "little snacks" as well?

Food Journal

Time of meal 1 - ________

Food eaten- ______________________

____

Drink - ______________________

Total Carb Grams -_____ **Total Calories -** ______

Time of meal 2 - ________

Food eaten- ______________________

____

Drink - ______________________

Total Carb grams - _____ **Total Calories -** ______

Time of meal 3 - ________

Food eaten- ______________________________

____

Drink - ______________________________

Total Carb Grams -_____ **Total Calories -** ______

Time of meal 4 - ________

Food eaten- ______________________________

____

Drink - ______________________________

Total Carb grams - _____ **Total Calories -** ______

Time of meal 5 - ________

Food eaten - ____

Drink -______________________________

Total Carb Grams -______ **Total Calories -** _______

And The Heart Says…

Tonight after you eat and are sitting down relaxing, take a heart rate and write it down here:

After dinner HR-________ **Time taken -** _______

Man these days go fast! Day 2 is done and up next is my favorite day: LEG DAY! Tomorrow's workout is very different and you'll be doing one legged exercises when you're used to using both legs. You're going to need all of your energy for this one so eat some good clean food, clear that beautiful mind of yours, and get that much needed sleep. See you tomorrow!

Round 2 – Day 3

Wow! Another Day 3 is here and let me tell you, it's a big one! Make sure you eat a good breakfast, take care of your pets, and get to work on time so nobody gets in trouble. Don't forget to smile; it's going to be another great day for you!

That One Thing

On Day 1 of this week, you wrote down one thing you thought could keep you from achieving what you want most from this program. Now, write down one thing you can do to make sure this doesn't happen.

To make sure I get what I want most out of this program, I'm going to…

____

Seeing I to Eye

Okay, I'm going to test you today. Find that secluded quiet place with no distractions and for 3 minutes visualize how you want to look in your bathing suit. Yep, this is a big one. Start with visualizing yourself at the beach or somewhere with water. Once you have this down, bring on you and your swimsuit. You can do it, just keep thinking good things.

Pre Game

It's very easy to get caught up in your work causing you to forget to do the things you need to do to prepare for your workouts. One thing you can do to help you stay on track is to set an alarm on your phone or write yourself a note and put it where you can see it every day. If you write a note, simply write these things down:

- Eat 1.5-2.5 hours before I exercise
- Drink plenty of water before I exercise
- Clear my mind, leave stress behind

Your Workout – See your workout log for today's workout

And the Heart Says…

While you're in bed tonight but before you go to sleep, take one more heart rate and record it here.

Pre Sleep HR - ______ Time taken - ______

Cleaning Your Plate

Do you know how many calories are in proteins, carbohydrates, and fats? If not, here you go:

- 1 gram of protein has 4 calories
- 1 gram of carbohydrates has 4 calories
- 1 gram of fat has 9 calories

Can you see why we should eat a low fat diet? Think about these differences in calories today as you fill in your food journal.

You Ate What???

Food Journal

Time of meal 1 - _________

Food eaten- ________________________________

____

Drink - ____________________________________

Total Carb Grams -______ Total Calories - ______

Time of meal 2 - _________

Food eaten- ____________________________________

____

Drink - _______________________________________

Total Carb grams - ______ Total Calories - _______

Time of meal 3 - ________

Food eaten- ______________________________

____

Drink - ______________________________

Total Carb Grams -______ **Total Calories -** _______

Time of meal 4 - ________

Food eaten- ______________________________

____

Drink - ______________________________

Total Carb grams - ______ **Total Calories -** _______

Time of meal 5 - ________

Food eaten - ____

Drink - ______________________________

Total Carb Grams -______ **Total Calories -** _______

You have reached the end of Day 3; what a day for you! It was leg day and you spent a lot of energy during your workout so make sure you get good clean food to eat for the remainder of your day, fill out that food journal, get something positive in your head, and go dream of something good. See you tomorrow!

Round 2, Day 4

Guess what? It's Day 4 again and that means a day off from working out for you. If you have been working out every day, this may seem weird to you and may take some getting used to but it will pay off for you in the long run. You have to let that body heal up so give it a break and enjoy this day off.

"Most of your success in fitness will come from what you do outside of your exercise program. The other parts, the most important parts, are what and when you eat, how well you sleep, how well you recuperate, and definitely what you think."

Bobby Whisnand

It Happened Just Like This!

I'll never forget how I felt that day last year when my PR agent said, "Bobby, it's time for you to write a book." I said, "Are you serious? I mean, I like to write but I'm not sure about a book." Of course that's all I thought about for the rest of that day and on the very next day, I started writing my first book titled "It's All Heart". After three months, I had finished the book and sent it off to the editor. All I could think about was whether or not she would like it, or send it back asking me to rewrite it. Well, I got my answer two days later in an email stating how much she liked it and how well I did for a first time author. That's all I needed because the very next day I started my second book, and six weeks later, I finished that one too. Just remember; at first things may seem insurmountable or overly challenging but you are capable of a lot more than you think. Stay tough, stay positive, and go get what you want out of life.

Which Way You Headed?

Last week you wrote down one long term goal about your fitness. Today, write that goal again and this time, write one short term (2 week) goal that will help you reach that long term goal.

My first long term (12 week) goal about my fitness is…

____

My first short term (2 week) goal to help me reach this long term goal is…

____

Seeing I to Eye

How's your vision these days? Are you getting better at picturing positive things about yourself? Today, take 3 minutes and visualize yourself doing an activity you love to do like anything outdoors, seeing a musical or play, going to a sporting event, etc. Don't forget to add all the good stuff like sounds, colors, the weather, etc.

Upper Management

On Day 2 you wrote a list of things you need to get done. Today, write down one thing from that list and write a plan to get it done.

Here's one thing from my list of things to get done from Day 2

____

Now here's my plan to get it done:

____

And the Heart Says…

At some point today, take and record your heart rate after you have been walking around from place to place like to and from your desk, to and from your car, or any other place that's a short light walk.

Short walk HR - ______ Time taken - ______

Cleaning Your Plate

Let's talk about fiber today. I know you've heard countless times about its importance but exactly what is it and what does it do for you? Common sources of fiber are fruits, vegetables, whole grains, and legumes and the fiber within these foods is non nutritious to your body. Your body uses it but not for energy or in any nutritious way. This is why many diets let you subtract fiber from your total carbohydrate intake. The main function of fiber, especially non soluble fiber, is to help your digestive system move things along as they should. You know what I'm talking about; do I need to explain any further? Good, I'm relieved. No joke intended.

You Ate What???

This is where things get very interesting because starting today, I want you to also journal how many grams of protein and fat you're consuming a day. This means you will be journaling total grams of carbs, proteins, and fats, and total calories consumed daily. Are you ready for this? Absolutely you are; here we go.

Food Journal

Time of meal 1 - _________

Food eaten- ____

Drink - __________________________________

Carbohydrates	**Protein**	**Fat**
Total carb grams -	Total protein grams -	Total fat grams -
Total Calories-		

Time of meal 2 - _________

Food eaten- ____

Drink - __________________________________

Carbohydrates	**Protein**	**Fat**
Total carb grams -	Total protein grams -	Total fat grams -
Total Calories-		

Time of meal 3 - _________

Food eaten- ____

Drink - __________________________________

Carbohydrates	**Protein**	**Fat**
Total crab grams -	Total protein grams -	Total fat grams -
Total Calories-		

Time of meal 4 - _________

Food eaten- ____

Drink - __________________________________

Carbohydrates	**Protein**	**Fat**
Total crab grams -	Total protein grams -	Total fat grams -
Total Calories-		

Time of meal 5 - _________

Food eaten- ____

Drink - __________________________________

Carbohydrates	**Protein**	**Fat**
Total crab grams -	Total protein grams -	Total fat grams -
Total Calories-		

Tomorrow is Friday and I've got a great back and bicep day planned for you. It's another unilateral day which as you have found out by now, definitely can be a challenge. Finish this day off in a great way by thinking positive, relaxing, and feeling good about what you've already accomplished with 12 Rounds. Now go dream BIG!

Round 2 - Day 5

Here we go! You get to show off a little today, are you ready? Are you telling me to shut up because it's too early for that stuff? That's okay; you'll love me later after you get done doing your Day 5 workout. Get some good food in you, make sure you feed, water, and hug those pets, and let's kick this thing off!

That One Thing

Last week you wrote down one person with whom you could share your experiences from this program. Make it a point today to let them know you are doing this program and you are counting on them for support. You can even show them this book to see what they think.

Seeing I to Eye

The reason I have you visualizing something every day is simple: I want you to get good at it and use it every day of your life because it will lead you to good places. Today, I want you to take 3-4 minutes and think back to a happy event in your life. Visualize that experience and just enjoy the moment. Once you're done, write a brief description here:

The happy event in my life I visualized today was ...

Pre Game

When was your last meal today? Are you timing your eating so that your food has had time to be digested and stored as energy for your workout? How much water have you drunk today?

Your Workout – See your workout log for today's workout.

And the Heart Says...

When you get home, sit down, rest for about a minute, take a heart rate, and write it down here.

Evening resting HR ______ Time taken - ______

Cleaning Your Plate

Do you know the difference between good and bad cholesterol? Just in case you don't, here are the two types of cholesterol and what makes them good or bad. The "good" cholesterol is called HDL which stands for high density lipoproteins and it's considered "good" cholesterol because it helps remove LDL (bad cholesterol) from the arteries. Sources of HDL are various fish, nuts, and olive oil. If you are not a fish lover, then fish oil supplements will suffice.

The "bad" cholesterol is called LDL which stands for low density lipids. LDL cholesterol is considered "bad" cholesterol because it contributes to plaque; a thick, hard deposit that can clog arteries and make them less flexible. This condition is known as atherosclerosis. Sources of LDL are animal products such as whole milk, butter, cream, ice cream, cheese, fatty meats, and vegetable oils such as palm and coconut. **Recommended limits of saturated fat intake are 10 percent of your total calories.**

There's one more thing I want you to know about cholesterol. Your body, more specifically your liver, makes just about all the cholesterol you need, so that's why you have to be very aware of how much cholesterol you are consuming with what you eat and drink. Watch out now, it can sneak up on you. Don't forget to get those numbers checked by your doctor.

You Ate What???

Since we are on the subject of fats and cholesterol, take a good look at how many grams of fat you are consuming for each meal. With 1 gram of fat equaling nine calories, it's easy to see how this can add up very fast. Yes, ice cream and chocolate count. Believe me; I wish they didn't either.

Food Journal

Time of meal 1 - _________

Food eaten- ____

Drink - __________________________________

Carbohydrates	**Protein**	**Fat**
Total crab grams -	Total protein grams -	Total fat grams -
Total Calories-		

Time of meal 2 - _________

Food eaten- ____

Drink - __________________________________

Carbohydrates	**Protein**	**Fat**
Total crab grams -	Total protein grams -	Total fat grams -
Total Calories-		

Time of meal 3 - _________

Food eaten- ____

Drink - __________________________________

Carbohydrates	**Protein**	**Fat**
Total crab grams -	Total protein grams -	Total fat grams -
Total Calories-		

Time of meal 4 - _________

Food eaten- ____

Drink - __________________________________

Carbohydrates	**Protein**	**Fat**
Total crab grams -	Total protein grams -	Total fat grams -
Total Calories-		

Time of meal 5 - _________

Food eaten- ____

Drink - __________________________________

Carbohydrates	**Protein**	**Fat**
Total crab grams -	Total protein grams -	Total fat grams -
Total Calories-		

Can you believe you're almost through the second round? Just wait; it keeps getting better and better. Tomorrow you have a cardio and abdominal workout which is different than last week so be ready for it. Make sure you're doing the things both before and after your workout that I list every day; these things make the biggest difference in how good your workouts really are. And don't forget; where the head goes the body follows so think positive. See you tomorrow!

Round 2- Day 6

Are you ready for a great day? Before we start, I want you to take a minute and think of how you feel physically. Do you feel rested, sore, fresh, or like you need more sleep? Either way, make a note below how you feel when you got up this morning.

This morning after I woke up, I felt…

____

Which Way You Headed?

Last week you wrote down one long term (12 week) goal about your career. Today, write that goal again and this time, write one short term (2 week) goal that will help you reach that long term goal.

My first long term (12 week) goal about my career is…

____

My first short term (2 week) goal that will help me reach this long term goal is…

____

Upper Management

Earlier this week you wrote down one thing that you need to get off your list of things to do. Did you get it done? If you did, that's awesome. Take another look at that list and start working on getting another thing checked off as well. If you didn't, write it again here and do your best to get it done before the start of next week.

That one thing I wrote down to get off my list of things to do is...

____

Seeing I to Eye

Today, right before you start your exercise routine; visualize yourself doing the first exercise perfectly. Take your time and see yourself taking 5 full seconds through the entire repetition including the pause at the top and bottom of each repetition. Also, see yourself being fit, strong, and full of endurance.

Pre Game

Get that body and mind ready to work out by eating the right foods at the right times, visualize yourself having a great workout, and make sure you are well hydrated before you start.

And the Heart Says...

You took a lot of heart rates today but that's a good thing. I want you to take one more so we can see how your heart is recovering from that awesome workout today. At some point this evening when you are relaxed, take another heart rate and record it here.

Post workout HR ______ Time taken - ______

Cleaning Your Plate

How much protein do you need in a day? This depends on several variables like your age, your activity level, your body weight, and your goals. The more active you are, the more protein you need, so this amount may change as your body changes. For me personally, I get 1.5 grams per pound of lean body weight which equals to around 250-280 grams of protein a day for me. But, I'm extremely active and my workouts are very demanding so I consume more protein than the average person. Here are the recommended daily amounts of protein from the Institute of Medicine:

- Teenage boys need up to 52 grams a day.
- Teenage girls need 46 grams a day.
- Adult men need about 56 grams a day.
- Adult women need about 46 grams a day (71 grams, if pregnant or breastfeeding)

You Ate What???

Are you leaving anything out of your food journal? The best thing to do is to take your journal with you when you eat and record it as soon as you're done. If not, things can get away from you during your day and you may forget exactly how much of a certain food you ate.

Food Journal

Time of meal 1 - _________

Food eaten- ____

Drink - __________________________________

Carbohydrates
Total crab grams -
Total Calories-

Protein
Total protein grams -

Fat
Total fat grams -

Time of meal 2 - _________

Food eaten- ____

Drink - __________________________________

Carbohydrates
Total crab grams -
Total Calories-

Protein
Total protein grams -

Fat
Total fat grams -

Time of meal 3 - _________

Food eaten- ____

Drink - __________________________________

Carbohydrates
Total crab grams -
Total Calories-

Protein
Total protein grams -

Fat
Total fat grams -

Time of meal 4 - _________

Food eaten- ____

Drink - __________________________________

Carbohydrates
Total crab grams -
Total Calories-

Protein
Total protein grams -

Fat
Total fat grams -

Time of meal 5 - _________

Food eaten- ____

Drink - __________________________________

Carbohydrates
Total crab grams -
Total Calories-

Protein
Total protein grams -

Fat
Total fat grams -

This was a great day for you and as you know, tomorrow you have the day off. Keep eating clean and don't forget your support when things get tough. Reach out to that person with whom you chose to share your progresses with 12 Rounds and let them know how you're doing. Rest up and I'll see you tomorrow. Another great day for you!

Round 2 - *Day 7*

It's your day off again, and you absolutely deserve it. What are your plans today? Whatever they are, enjoy yourself; you've definitely earned it. Just like last week, I have put a place for you to record a heart rate and a food journal just in case you wanted to log your food and drink. Again, you don't have to, but it's here if you choose to do so. Great job this week, I'll see you tomorrow for Round 3!

Day 7 HR ______ Time taken - ______

Food Journal

Time of meal 1 - _________

Food eaten- ____

Drink - __________________________________

Carbohydrates
Total crab grams -
Total Calories-

Protein
Total protein grams -

Fat
Total fat grams -

Time of meal 2 - _________

Food eaten- ____

Drink - __________________________________

Carbohydrates
Total crab grams -
Total Calories-

Protein
Total protein grams -

Fat
Total fat grams -

Time of meal 3 - _________

Food eaten- ____

Drink - __________________________________

Carbohydrates
Total crab grams -
Total Calories-

Protein
Total protein grams -

Fat
Total fat grams -

Time of meal 4 - _________

Food eaten- ____

Drink - __________________________________

Carbohydrates
Total crab grams -

Protein
Total protein grams -

Fat
Total fat grams -

Total Calories-

Time of meal 5 - _________

Food eaten- ____

Drink - __________________________________

Carbohydrates
Total crab grams -

Protein
Total protein grams -

Fat
Total fat grams -

Total Calories-

Round 3 – Flipping the Script – A Different Approach

Are you ready for Round 3? I know you are because you went through Rounds 1 and 2 like a champ. As I told you during the introduction of this book, every round you do is considerably different than all the other rounds and Round 3 is absolutely no exception. I really flip the script on you this week by doing two very different things in your workouts. The first thing that changes is you will be using heavier resistance and the second and biggest difference of all…you'll be doing all exercises in reverse order from what you did on your first two weeks. Oh yes; how's that for a change? This is where things start to really take off for you and your body so make sure you follow this program exactly as I show you so you'll knock this thing out of the park.

Don't forget to take a look at the Appendix in the back of your workout log so you can see how the weights change when you go in reverse; it's a really big difference, especially toward the end of your workouts. Don't say I didn't warn you.

The number one cause of disability in the United States is joint pain and arthritis affecting over 100 million people. That's more people than are affected by cancer, heart disease, and diabetes combined

Day 1

It Happened Just Like This!

After I finished writing my first book, I immediately started thinking about a title for my second book and within one day, I knew exactly what it was going to be. I titled my second book "***A Body To Die For: The Painful Truth about Exercise.***" The subject of this book is how millions of people are taking years off their lives by destroying their joints and prematurely aging their bodies by exercising incorrectly. My book points out that as a nation, we have a pandemic of joint pain where over 1/3 of our population is affected by chronic pain and arthritis, and it's not only our inactive and unhealthy populations that are contributing; it's also our overactive populations and the way they are exercising. Check out these statistics on our nation's problem with joint pain:

- With the aging of the U.S. population, the prevalence of doctor-diagnosed arthritis is expected to increase in the coming decades. By the year 2030, an estimated 67 million (25% of the projected total adult population) adults aged 18 years and older will have doctor-diagnosed arthritis, compared with the 50 million adults in 2007–2009.
- **The number of total knee replacements performed in the U.S. will leap by 673% reaching 3.48 million by the year 2030.** This is according to a study by the American Academy of Orthopaedic Surgery in Chicago.
- Hip replacements will increase by 174% to 572,000 by 2030.
- **Back pain is the leading cause of disability in Americans under 45 years old.**
- In addition, back pain leaves about 2.4 million Americans chronically disabled and another 2.4 million temporarily disabled.
- And, if that wasn't enough, about 60 - 80% of the adult U.S. population has low back pain, and it is the second most common reason people go to the doctor.

So what do think, pretty scary huh? This is the exact reason I designed 12 Rounds; to teach you how to build a strong well balanced and healthy body by exercising the one right way so you'll keep your joints healthy and stay mobile for the rest of your life.

That One Thing

Today during your workout, make sure you are going slow and using controlled movement with every single repetition you do. Every rep should take you 4-5 seconds with a complete pause at the top and bottom. As long as you do all exercises in this way, you will not only avoid joint damage, you will build joint health which will last you a very long time. Go Slow, I'm watching you!

Seeing I to Eye

Go to that quiet place and for 3-4 minutes visualize whatever you want; as long as it's positive. Go ahead; it's your choice today. Just be sure to be very specific with what you are seeing.

Write down what you visualized here:

____

Pre Game

Are you ready for your workout today? More specifically, is your body and mind ready?

Don't forget to take a look at the appendix of my workout in the back of your workout log so you can get an idea of how much weight you're going to need today. Remember, everything is in REVERSE!

Your Workout – See your workout log for today's workout

And the Heart Says…

Tonight when you are lying in bed and before you go to sleep, take one more heart rate and write it down here.

Pre Sleep HR - ______ Time taken - ______

Cleaning Your Plate

Look at a label on something you drink and find how many total servings are in the container. Now multiply total calories by the number of servings. While you're at it, do the same for the simple sugars in your drink. If it's water, great job; no homework for you!

You Ate What???

Today we're going to add a few things to your food journal. I want you to start journaling the carbohydrate breakdown in everything you eat and drink. Here is how most carbohydrates are broken down on food and drink labels:

- Total Carbs
- Dietary Fiber
- Sugar

If you remember, in Round 2 I had you take a look at the carbohydrate breakdown and I showed you how to figure out how many of the total carbohydrates are complex. All you have to do is add the sugars and the fibers together and subtract that number from the total carbs. This will give you the number of complex carbs in a particular food or drink. Remember, fiber is a complex carb but it's non nutritious to your body. It takes a little more time but it will help you tremendously in understanding how to eat better for your needs.

Food Journal

Time of meal 1 - _________

Food eaten- ____

Drink - ________________________

Carbohydrates	**Protein**	**Fat**
Total carb grams -	Total protein grams -	Total fat grams -
Total fiber grams -		
Total sugar grams -		
Total complex grams -		
Total calories of meal -	**cal**	

Time of meal 2 - _________

Food eaten- ____

Drink - ________________________

Carbohydrates	**Protein**	**Fat**
Total carb grams -	Total protein grams -	Total fat grams -
Total fiber grams -		
Total sugar grams -		
Total complex grams -		
Total calories of meal -	**cal**	

Time of meal 3 - _________

Food eaten- ____

Drink - ________________________

Carbohydrates	**Protein**	**Fat**
Total carb grams -	Total protein grams -	Total fat grams -
Total fiber grams -		
Total sugar grams -		
Total complex grams -		
Total calories of meal -	**cal**	

Time of meal 4 - _________

Food eaten- ____

Drink - ________________________

Carbohydrates	**Protein**	**Fat**
Total carb grams -	Total protein grams -	Total fat grams -
Total fiber grams -		
Total sugar grams -		
Total complex grams -		
Total calories of meal -	**cal**	

Time of meal 5 - _________

Food eaten- ____

Drink - ________________________

Carbohydrates	**Protein**	**Fat**
Total carb grams -	Total protein grams -	Total fat grams -
Total fiber grams -		
Total sugar grams -		
Total complex grams -		
Total calories of meal -	**cal**	

There you have it; Day 1 of Round 3 is in the books. What do you think about the "reverse" workout today? I told you it was a big difference. The idea is to make your body respond to different stimulus in exercise by incorporating different muscles in different ways. This is how you build a strong well balanced body and keep it interesting as well. You know the drill; eat up, rest up, relax, think about good things, and go dream big! See you tomorrow!

Round 3, Day 2

You've got a great start to Rounds 3; let's keep it going with an awesome core and cardio day. One thing I want you to start thinking about is your level of soreness you're having on the days after your workouts. If you're having mild to moderate soreness that last for 48-72 hours, that's where you need to be. If you are having severe soreness or your soreness is lasting for more than 72 hours, I want you to reduce the amount of weight you are using within your workouts. If you aren't having any soreness, and your form and technique are perfect, go ahead and increase your weights, but just by a little bit.

Which Way You Headed?

At this point, you have one long term goal about something other than fitness. Write that goal again and in addition, write one more long term (10 week) goal about something other than fitness.

My first long term (12 week) goal about something other than my fitness is…

____

My second long term (10 week) goal about something other than my fitness is…

____

Seeing I to Eye

If you could go anywhere in the world, where would you go? Write that place down here and at some point today, visualize yourself there. Be sure to add the weather, sounds, other people, animals, and anything else that goes with your trip.

The one place in the world I want to go to the most is…

Upper Management

One of the biggest ways stress gets the better of us is when we are late for a meeting, work, appointment, or something else important. Today, think of one thing you can do to start managing your time better like making a schedule and going over it daily, getting up a little earlier each morning, or using reminders. Once you got it, write it down here:

One thing I'm going to start doing to manage my time better is…

Pre Game

Get that body and mind ready; you've got a heck of a core and cardio workout today.

Your Workout – See your workout log for today's workout

Cleaning Your Plate

Why are vegetable so good for us?

We all know vegetables are good for us but exactly why? Vegetables are our best source of vitamins and minerals, they are full of fiber, and most of them are extremely low in simple sugars. They are one of the cleanest forms of nutrition we have because most of them are very low in fat, and the fat that is found in vegetables is much healthier than the fat found in animal products. Vegetables are filling and our bodies can use them very fast for energy and other body functions. I always tell my clients to make sure that half of their plate is made up of vegetables for each meal.

You Ate What???

Take a look at your journal at the end of the day and see how much of your diet is made up of vegetables. You should shoot for 4-5 servings of vegetables a day. Oh yea, fruit is good too; we will talk about it coming up soon. I'm also going to add a great resource for you to start taking a real close look at the foods you're eating and exactly what's in them. This is a list of all foods, their calories, and how much carbohydrates, proteins, and fats they have in them. Take a look; it's a great way to learn.

//ndb.nal.usda.gov/ndb/search/list

Food Journal

Time of meal 1 - _________

Food eaten- ____

Drink - ________________________

Carbohydrates	**Protein**	**Fat**
Total crab grams -	Total protein grams -	Total fat grams -
Total fiber grams -		
Total sugar grams -		
Total complex grams -		
Total calories of meal -	**cal**	

Time of meal 2 - _________

Food eaten- ____

Drink - ________________________

Carbohydrates	**Protein**	**Fat**
Total crab grams -	Total protein grams -	Total fat grams -
Total fiber grams -		
Total sugar grams -		
Total complex grams -		
Total calories of meal -	**cal**	

Time of meal 3 - _________

Food eaten- ____

Drink - ________________________

Carbohydrates	**Protein**	**Fat**
Total crab grams -	Total protein grams -	Total fat grams -
Total fiber grams -		
Total sugar grams -		
Total complex grams -		
Total calories of meal -	**cal**	

Time of meal 4 - _________

Food eaten- ____

Drink - ________________________

Carbohydrates	**Protein**	**Fat**
Total crab grams -	Total protein grams -	Total fat grams -
Total fiber grams -		
Total sugar grams -		
Total complex grams -		
Total calories of meal -	**cal**	

Time of meal 5 - _________

Food eaten- ____

Drink - ________________________

Carbohydrates	**Protein**	**Fat**
Total crab grams -	Total protein grams -	Total fat grams -
Total fiber grams -		
Total sugar grams -		
Total complex grams -		
Total calories of meal -	**cal**	

And The Heart Says…

Tonight after you eat and are sitting down relaxing, take a heart rate and write it down here:

After dinner HR-________ **Time taken -** ______

It's been another great day for you and it's time to relax. The only thing I want you to do tonight before you call it a day is to take a look at the workout you're doing tomorrow. In addition, take a look at the same workout in the appendix in the back of your workout log and get an idea of how your weights are going to change tomorrow because it's reverse week. It's Leg Day tomorrow and you'll be finishing with the hardest exercises so get your mind ready. Okay, that's enough; I'll shut up so you can take it easy. Rest up; you're going to need it!

Round 3 – Day 3

Are you ready for LEG DAY? I promise you a very different experience today, but it's going to be awesome! Let's go knock this out!

That One Thing

Today while you're warming up for your workout and in between your sets, take a look around the gym and see if there is anyone going as slow and controlled with their exercises as you are. I can already tell you what you're going to find.

Seeing I to Eye

Today, get in that quiet place and spend 3-4 minutes visualizing how you want to feel physically like having more energy, thinking clearly, being confident in your appearance, or just being content with your life. Make sure you clear your mind of any negative or stressful thoughts before you start your visualization; this will help you see things clearly.

Pre Game

As a reminder, here's that list of things to do before all of your workouts.

- Schedule your workouts just like a work appointment
- Make sure you eat 1.5-2 hours before you exercise
- Review your workout so you know what to expect
- Drink plenty of water before you workout
- If you are taking supplements, make sure you have them with you and take them at the right times
- Take a few minutes before you workout and clear your mind

Your Workout – See your workout log for today's workout

And the Heart Says…

At some point today while you're sitting around, take a heart rate and write it down here. Are you noticing a drop in your daily heart rates other than the heart rates you take when you exercise?

Resting HR - ______ Time taken - ______

Cleaning Your Plate

The American Heart Association says that we should limit our daily sodium intake to no more than 1500 mgs a day. This isn't much, and if you want to know what 1500 mgs of sodium looks like, fill a teaspoon of salt ¾ of the way up and you'll have it. See, I told you it wasn't much. Start thinking about your sodium intake because coming up soon, you'll be adding it to your food journal.

You Ate What???

You're doing great with your journal. Just remember, the more specific and detailed you fill out your journal, the better you're going to do at cleaning your plate.

Food Journal

Time of meal 1 - _________

Food eaten- ____

Drink - __________________________

Carbohydrates	**Protein**	**Fat**
Total crab grams -	Total protein grams -	Total fat grams -
Total fiber grams -		
Total sugar grams -		
Total complex grams -		
Total calories of meal -	**cal**	

Time of meal 2 - _________

Food eaten- ____

Drink - ________________________

Carbohydrates	**Protein**	**Fat**
Total crab grams -	Total protein grams -	Total fat grams -
Total fiber grams -		
Total sugar grams -		
Total complex grams -		
Total calories of meal -	**cal**	

Time of meal 3 - _________

Food eaten- ____

Drink - ________________________

Carbohydrates	**Protein**	**Fat**
Total crab grams -	Total protein grams -	Total fat grams -
Total fiber grams -		
Total sugar grams -		
Total complex grams -		
Total calories of meal -	**cal**	

Time of meal 4 - _________

Food eaten- ____

Drink - ________________________

Carbohydrates	**Protein**	**Fat**
Total crab grams -	Total protein grams -	Total fat grams -
Total fiber grams -		
Total sugar grams -		
Total complex grams -		
Total calories of meal -	**cal**	

Time of meal 5 - _________

Food eaten- ____

Drink - ________________________

Carbohydrates	**Protein**	**Fat**
Total crab grams -	Total protein grams -	Total fat grams -
Total fiber grams -		
Total sugar grams -		
Total complex grams -		
Total calories of meal -	**cal**	

Another good thing about leg day is the fact that you will get some good sleep. When you train your legs, your body expends the most energy and therefore tells you it needs rest and recuperation. Give it what it needs and it will give you what you need.

Great job today; I'll see you tomorrow for Day 4.

Round 3, Day 4

What's up Champ? Did you rest those legs last night? There are a lot of people out there who over train their bodies because they neglect to take days off and fully recuperate. Even if someone is over training just one muscle group like legs, their entire body will be affected in a negative way. This is your day off from exercise; make sure you keep it that way.

"Some of the simplest things a person can do to better their health are also the most common things neglected by many people, and the most damaging."

Bobby Whisnand

It Happened Just Like This!

There's one thing I hear a lot in the gym and its one thing I wish I didn't hear at all. One of those conversations I overheard was between a trainer and his client and it went just like this: The client said, "I'm not sure I should work out today, my legs hurt so much from our workout yesterday, I can barely walk and my knee is swollen." The trainer replied "Oh you'll be fine, you need to work your legs again so the soreness will leave." The client then said "but my doctor told me if my knee swelled up, I should not exercise on it at all and ice it." The trainer responded, "If it gets too bad we will just lighten your weight and keep going."

This should NEVER happen, but it's a common occurrence in the training industry.

First of all, you should never get so sore you can't walk, and secondly, if you have swelling anywhere, something is wrong and you need to stop and go see your doctor. Be very careful of the fitness advice you receive because from my experience in this business, much of it is incorrect and harmful.

Which Way You Headed?

Last week you wrote down one long term goal about fitness. Today, write down that first goal again and in addition, write a second long term (10 week) goal about your fitness.

My first long term (12 week) goal about my fitness is...

My second long term (10 week) goal about my fitness is...

Seeing I to Eye

Last week you visualized yourself doing something in which you have little confidence. Try this again today and this time shoot for 5 minutes and concentrate on adding sounds, colors, and other people responding positively to what you're doing or saying. See Your Success!

Upper Management

It's time to clear the air. Today I want you to take a moment and think about someone with whom things aren't so good between the two of you. Maybe it was a misunderstanding or just one of those touchy subjects, but these things cause stress when they aren't resolved. Swallow your pride, open your heart, and call that person and get things back on track. Even if you call to just say hello, this could be the one thing that could get you two back on the right track. Go ahead, make that call.

No Workout Today! – Take this day and catch up in places where you might be behind. Also, keep your diet the same and make sure you record everything in your food journal.

And the Heart Says…

Take at least one heart rate today whenever you want. Just make sure you write down when and under what circumstances you took it.

Today I took my heart rate when I was… ______________________________________

Day 4 HR - ______ Time taken - ______

Cleaning Your Plate

If you are trying to shed a few pounds, one of the best ways to do this is to greatly reduce your carbohydrates across the day, especially with your dinner. Instead of eating foods like pasta, rice, potatoes, and bread, replace those with green leafy vegetables. I don't suggest you completely cut out all complex carbs because you need those for energy, but just reduce the amount you eat. You'll also want to greatly reduce or completely avoid the simple carbohydrates like sweeteners and foods that have a lot of "sugars" in them. You can eat some fruit during the day but other than that, stay away from the sweet stuff.

You Ate What???

How are you doing with the newly added carbohydrate breakdowns? One thing is for sure; you're going to become very aware of just how much of each carbohydrate you're consuming, and this is one of the biggest keys to controlling and maintaining a healthy body weight. Keep it up; you're doing great!

Food Journal

Time of meal 1 - _________

Food eaten- ____

Drink - _______________________

Carbohydrates	**Protein**	**Fat**
Total carb grams -	Total protein grams -	Total fat grams -
Total fiber grams -		
Total sugar grams -		
Total complex grams -		
Total calories of meal -	**cal**	

Time of meal 2 - _________

Food eaten- ____

Drink - ________________________

Carbohydrates	**Protein**	**Fat**
Total crab grams -	Total protein grams -	Total fat grams -
Total fiber grams -		
Total sugar grams -		
Total complex grams -		
Total calories of meal -	**cal**	

Time of meal 3 - _________

Food eaten- ____

Drink - ________________________

Carbohydrates	**Protein**	**Fat**
Total crab grams -	Total protein grams -	Total fat grams -
Total fiber grams -		
Total sugar grams -		
Total complex grams -		
Total calories of meal -	**cal**	

Time of meal 4 - _________

Food eaten- ____

Drink - ________________________

Carbohydrates	**Protein**	**Fat**
Total crab grams -	Total protein grams -	Total fat grams -
Total fiber grams -		
Total sugar grams -		
Total complex grams -		
Total calories of meal -	**cal**	

Time of meal 5 - _________

Food eaten- ____

Drink - ________________________

Carbohydrates	**Protein**	**Fat**
Total crab grams -	Total protein grams -	Total fat grams -
Total fiber grams -		
Total sugar grams -		
Total complex grams -		
Total calories of meal -	**cal**	

How did you feel on your day off from working out? Remember, most of your success in fitness will come from what you do outside of your exercise routine and that includes eating right, sleeping, managing your stress, and…taking days off from exercise. We just took a day off, now it's up to you to eat some good food, sleep well, and keep positive things in that brain of yours. Tomorrow is going to be a great day for you; put that in your head and make it so!

Round 3 - Day 5

Hey you! How did you sleep last night? If you are having trouble getting to sleep or getting quality sleep, try using what you have learned with your daily visualization. Also, make sure you are fully relaxed when you go to bed and clear your mind of worries. Here we go with Day 5 which as you know by now is back and bicep day. It's a heavy reverse workout so be ready to work.

That One Thing

During your workout today, concentrate on the targeted muscle or muscles for each exercise and picture them working as you workout. For example: When you are doing the seated row, visualize your back muscles flexing as you pull, and stretching as you release. Remember, GO SLOW, always have good form, and don't watch what others are doing; you know why.

Seeing I to Eye

At the end of today, take a few minutes and think about the workout you did earlier. Visualize a few of the exercises you did and see yourself doing them with full control, perfect from, and technique. Remember, where the head goes, the body will follow.

Pre Game

Are you getting into the habit of doing your pre workout things? Make these things just as much a part of your workout as the actual workout itself.

Your Workout – See your workout log for today's workout.

And the Heart Says…

Some time tonight after you eat dinner and when you have been relaxing for an hour or so, take and record a heart rate.

Evening resting HR ______ Time taken - ______

Cleaning Your Plate

There's one thing we haven't talked about much up to this point, and that's how much water you're drinking a day. A standard recommendation you will often see is to drink 64 ounces a day. However, this varies according to your body weight, how active you are, your current fitness level, and the temperature outside. In my opinion, the 64 ounce mark is a minimum amount and if you are working out, especially with this program, I would bump that number up to at least 90 -120 ounces a day. The key thing about drinking water is to never get to a point where you are thirsty, and that means drinking enough throughout your day and increasing the amounts during activity or workouts.

You Ate What???

For now, I'm going to keep your food journal the same but next week, I'm going to add one small thing to your journal. Do you have any idea what it is? Here's a hint: It's nothing you eat.

Food Journal

Time of meal 1 - _________

Food eaten- ____

Drink - ________________________

Carbohydrates	**Protein**	**Fat**
Total crab grams -	Total protein grams -	Total fat grams -
Total fiber grams -		
Total sugar grams -		
Total complex grams -		
Total calories of meal -	**cal**	

Time of meal 2 - _________

Food eaten- ____

Drink - ________________________

Carbohydrates	**Protein**	**Fat**
Total crab grams -	Total protein grams -	Total fat grams -
Total fiber grams -		
Total sugar grams -		
Total complex grams -		
Total calories of meal -	**cal**	

Time of meal 3 - _________

Food eaten- ____

Drink - ________________________

Carbohydrates	**Protein**	**Fat**
Total crab grams -	Total protein grams -	Total fat grams -
Total fiber grams -		
Total sugar grams -		
Total complex grams -		
Total calories of meal -	**cal**	

Time of meal 4 - _________

Food eaten- ____

Drink - ________________________

Carbohydrates
Total crab grams -
Total fiber grams -
Total sugar grams -
Total complex grams -

Protein
Total protein grams -

Fat
Total fat grams -

Total calories of meal - **cal**

Time of meal 5 - _________

Food eaten- ____

Drink - ________________________

Carbohydrates
Total crab grams -
Total fiber grams -
Total sugar grams -
Total complex grams -

Protein
Total protein grams -

Fat
Total fat grams -

Total calories of meal - **cal**

How did you do on your workout today? That reverse day is really different isn't it? You have one more workout tomorrow and then you get another day off. Before then, make sure you are doing the things you need to do to recuperate from your workouts by eating the right foods at the right times, getting good quality sleep, and keeping that mind positive. Go dream BIG! I'll see you tomorrow!

Round 3 - Day 6

Are you ready for some core and cardio? I guess we'll soon find out. Before we get going, I want you to make a quick note on how you feel this morning. Are you sore, tired, full of energy, hungry, excited, etc? Write how you're feeling right here:

____

Which Way You Headed?

On Round 1 you wrote down one long term (12 week) goal about your career. Today, write that goal again and in addition, write down a second long term (10 week) goal about your career.

My first long term (12 week) goal about my career is -

____

My second long term (10 week) goal about my career is…

____

Upper Management

Last week you wrote down one thing that you need to get off your list of things to do and I'm assuming you got it done. Go back to Day 2 of Round 2 and write that list again here. This time pick another thing to get off your list and make a plan to get it done before the next round.

These are the things I need to get done to lighten my load:

1. ______________________________ 7. ______________________________

2. ______________________________ 8. ______________________________

3. ______________________________ 9. ______________________________

4. ______________________________ 10. ______________________________

5. ______________________________ 11. ______________________________

6. ______________________________ 12. ______________________________

Another thing I am going to get off my list of things to do is…

____

Seeing I to Eye

Take 3-4 minutes right before you start your workout and visualize the first core exercise. See yourself doing 5-6 reps of that exercise slowly, in control, and with perfect form. Watch that neck!

Pre Game

Keep up the good work by making sure you're ready to exercise and don't forget to clear your mind and leave stress behind.

Your Workout – See your workout log for today's workout.

And the Heart Says…

At some point this evening when you are relaxed, take another heart rate and record it here.

Post workout/evening HR ______ Time taken - ______

Cleaning Your Plate

One question about nutrition I get asked often is… *"Is it bad to eat right before I go to bed?"*

The answer is…It depends on what you're eating and what your body weight goals are. If your goal is to lose some weight, it's okay to eat right before you go to bed on two conditions: The first condition is if it has been 2-3 hours since you last ate, and the second condition is if you only eat a small amount of lean protein and/or a non starchy vegetable like something green and leafy. You absolutely want to stay away from complex carbohydrates, simple sugars, and fats right before you go to bed. If you do eat these things, there's a high likely hood your body will store these as body fat because you are at rest and there's no place for that energy to be spent.

On the other hand, if you are trying to gain weight, it's not only okay, it can be beneficial for you to eat right before you go to bed, but apply the same principle above with the exception of adding a very small amount of clean complex carbohydrates to the mix. The important thing to do is to record everything you eat and drink so you can see what effect your diet is having on your body.

You Ate What???

Food Journal

Time of meal 1 - _________

Food eaten- ____

Drink - ________________________

Carbohydrates	**Protein**	**Fat**
Total crab grams -	Total protein grams -	Total fat grams -
Total fiber grams -		
Total sugar grams -		
Total complex grams -		
Total calories of meal -	**cal**	

Time of meal 2 - _________

Food eaten- ____

Drink - ________________________

Carbohydrates	**Protein**	**Fat**
Total crab grams -	Total protein grams -	Total fat grams -
Total fiber grams -		
Total sugar grams -		
Total complex grams -		
Total calories of meal -	**cal**	

Time of meal 3 - _________

Food eaten- ____

Drink - ________________________

Carbohydrates	**Protein**	**Fat**
Total crab grams -	Total protein grams -	Total fat grams -
Total fiber grams -		
Total sugar grams -		
Total complex grams -		
Total calories of meal -	**cal**	

Time of meal 4 - _________

Food eaten- ____

Drink - ________________________

Carbohydrates	**Protein**	**Fat**
Total crab grams -	Total protein grams -	Total fat grams -
Total fiber grams -		
Total sugar grams -		
Total complex grams -		
Total calories of meal -	**cal**	

Time of meal 5 - _________

Food eaten- ____

Drink - ________________________

Carbohydrates	**Protein**	**Fat**
Total crab grams -	Total protein grams -	Total fat grams -
Total fiber grams -		
Total sugar grams -		
Total complex grams -		
Total calories of meal -	**cal**	

At the very beginning of this book, I told you that succeeding in fitness is a lot more than exercising and eating well. You have to set goals, prepare for and recuperate after exercise, manage your stress, and learn to be happy. This is exactly why we do these things in this book. If you keep up with it and give your best efforts, you'll make more progress than you ever have in all parts of your life. Keep up the hard work and I'll see you tomorrow!

Round 3 - Day 7

There's nothing like a day off to do what you want without a plan or agenda. The only things I want you to do is relax, have fun, think positive, and enjoy your progress with 12 Rounds. Just like the last two weeks, I have a place for you to take and record a heart rate and journal your food, but you absolutely don't have to do either one. Enjoy your day, and I'll be waiting for you tomorrow to start Round 4; it's going to be a good one!

Day 7 HR ______ **Time taken -** ______

Food Journal

Time of meal 1 - _________

Food eaten- ____

Drink - ________________________

Carbohydrates	**Protein**	**Fat**
Total crab grams -	Total protein grams -	Total fat grams -
Total fiber grams -		
Total sugar grams -		
Total complex grams -		
Total calories of meal -	**cal**	

Time of meal 2 - _________

Food eaten- ____

Drink - ________________________

Carbohydrates	**Protein**	**Fat**
Total crab grams -	Total protein grams -	Total fat grams -
Total fiber grams -		
Total sugar grams -		
Total complex grams -		
Total calories of meal -	**cal**	

Time of meal 3 - _________

Food eaten- ____

Drink - ________________________

Carbohydrates	**Protein**	**Fat**
Total crab grams -	Total protein grams -	Total fat grams -
Total fiber grams -		
Total sugar grams -		
Total complex grams -		
Total calories of meal -	**cal**	

Time of meal 4 - _________

Food eaten- ____

Drink - ________________________

Carbohydrates	**Protein**	**Fat**
Total crab grams -	Total protein grams -	Total fat grams -
Total fiber grams -		
Total sugar grams -		
Total complex grams -		
Total calories of meal -	**cal**	

Time of meal 5 - ________

Food eaten- ____

Drink - ________________________

Carbohydrates	**Protein**	**Fat**
Total crab grams -	Total protein grams -	Total fat grams -
Total fiber grams -		
Total sugar grams -		
Total complex grams -		
Total calories of meal -	**cal**	

Round 4 – Your Life, Your Terms

Day 1

I can't believe we are already starting Round 4! Although each round is considerably different, there will be some things that are similar but they'll always have a twist. We're going to start Round 4 off with a reverse light week, and boy I'm telling you; it's going to be a barn burner. In terms of the other things you're going to do like setting goals and managing your stress, we're going to be more proactive during this round, but I know you're ready for it. Let's turn up the heat, burn some body fat, keep your mind headed in the right direction, and have some fun! Here you go: Round 4!

"Yoda had it right; there's an awful lot of wanting, trying, and "meaning to" in this world; what we need is a lot more people doing." ***Bobby Whisnand***

It Happened Just Like This!

I've got a great story for you to kick off Round 4. It was 1994 and I had just given my notice at the gym where I started my personal training career. When I gave my notice, my boss told me I would never make it as an independent personal trainer. I thought, "Just you wait and see buddy." That very day I went into as many businesses as I could, introduced myself, and gave them a flyer. The flyer simply said "Bobby Whisnand, Cooper Clinic Certified Personal Trainer offers body fat testing to your entire company, free of charge." I had my beeper number on there too (yes, I said beeper) because I had no mobile phone. I did this on my lunch break, after work, and on my days off and I only stopped after two weeks because I had scheduled 26 different companies for body fat testing. Not bad huh? But the better news was, I picked up 16 personal training clients and I never looked back.

I guess you could say I took a chance going out on my own, but what I really did was do something proactive and pursue something I loved to do. By doing so, I put myself in a place where I was happy, a place where I could accomplish big things, and a place where I could help others do the same. And just like the song says, I did it my way.

That One Thing

For your first day of Round 4, be proactive today and do one thing that will improve your life like eating a very clean meal, helping someone without being asked, turn a negative situation into a positive one, or anything else that moves you forward. Once you know what it is you're going to do, write it down and go to it.

The one proactive thing I'm going to do today to improve my life is…

____

Seeing I to Eye

Find that quiet place and for 4-5 minutes, visualize yourself being successful with your career. It can be finishing a project, getting a raise, meeting your quota, making a sale, or anything positive about your career.

Write down what you visualized here:

____

Pre Game

Are you ready for your workout? Are you sure? Okay then, go get it done.

Your Workout – See your workout log for today's workout

And the Heart Says…

Tonight when you are lying in bed and before you go to sleep, take one more heart rate and write it down here.

Pre Sleep HR - ______ Time taken - ______

Cleaning Your Plate

How is the sugar in fruit different than table sugar, most sweeteners, baked sweets, and desserts? First of all, I am talking about simple sugars; the sugars which are broken down very quickly by your body and are in turn used up very quickly. The main difference between the simple sugar in fruit and the simple sugar in most sweeteners, baked sweets, and desserts is a matter of one being a natural sugar and the other being a processed sugar. Can you guess which one is the natural sugar? That's right; the sugar in fruit is the natural sugar as long as it's in its whole, natural, and raw state. But be aware, when fruit is converted into fruit juices, it is often and most times processed and stripped of many of its original nutrition. These are the sugars you want to avoid as much as possible and the only way to know is to read the ingredients on food and drink labels. You got me? Good, enough of that.

You Ate What???

I've got great news for you! The only thing we're going to add to your food journal this week is the amount of water you're drinking throughout your day. No big deal right? Let's do it.

Food Journal

Time of meal 1 - _________

Food eaten- ____

Drink - ________________________

Carbohydrates	**Protein**	**Fat**
Total crab grams -	Total protein grams -	Total fat grams -
Total fiber grams -		
Total sugar grams -		
Total complex grams -		

Total calories of meal - **cal**
Total ounces of water with meal - **ounces**

Time of meal 2 - _________

Food eaten- ____

Drink - ________________________

Carbohydrates	**Protein**	**Fat**
Total crab grams -	Total protein grams -	Total fat grams -
Total fiber grams -		
Total sugar grams -		
Total complex grams -		

Total calories of meal - **cal**
Total ounces of water with meal - **ounces**

Time of meal 3 (Lunch) - _________

Food eaten- ____

Drink - ________________________

Carbohydrates	**Protein**	**Fat**
Total crab grams -	Total protein grams -	Total fat grams -
Total fiber grams -		
Total sugar grams -		
Total complex grams -		

Total calories of meal - **cal**
Total ounces of water with meal - **ounces**

Time of meal 4 - _________

Food eaten- ____

Drink - ________________________

Carbohydrates	**Protein**	**Fat**
Total crab grams -	Total protein grams -	Total fat grams -
Total fiber grams -		
Total sugar grams -		
Total complex grams -		

Total calories of meal - **cal**
Total ounces of water with meal - **ounces**

Time of meal 5 - _________

Food eaten- ____

Drink - ________________________

Carbohydrates	**Protein**	**Fat**
Total crab grams -	Total protein grams -	Total fat grams -
Total fiber grams -		
Total sugar grams -		
Total complex grams -		

Total calories of meal - **cal**
Total ounces of water with meal - **ounces**

Total ounces of water with meals - ounces
Total ounces of water during workout - ounces
Total ounces of water outside meals - ounces
Total ounces of water today - ounces

Great job today; you nailed it! Day 2 of Round 4 is up next; are you ready for some core and cardio? Rest up and put a smile on that face; you're well on your way to where you want to be. See you tomorrow!

Round 4, Day 2

Good Morning Champ! Are you ready for another great day? Here it comes!

Which Way You Headed?

At this point, you have two long term goals about something other than fitness. Today, write those goals again and while you're at it, write down how you think you're doing in reaching these two goals.

My first long term (12 week) goal about something other than fitness is…

____

With this first long term goal, I think I'm…

____

My second long term (10 week) goal about something other than fitness is…

____

With this second long term goal, I think I'm…

____

Seeing I to Eye

Today I want you to think about one talent you wish you had, like being able to play professional sports, singing, playing an instrument, public speaking, being a dancing machine, etc. Once you have it, take 3-4 minutes and visualize yourself using this talent and write it down here as well.

The talent I wish I had but the one I can definitely see myself doing is…

____

Upper Management

Make sure you are getting good quality sleep. Before you go to sleep tonight or take a nap today, try to relax as much as possible, do your best to clear your mind of everything from that day, and picture being somewhere peaceful like on the beach, in the mountains, or anywhere you would like to be. It's your mind and your life; don't let anything or anyone else control it.

Pre Game

Get ready because your workout is coming up soon; you know the drill.

Your Workout – See your workout log for today's workout.

Cleaning Your Plate

Here's a very popular and debated topic for us to discuss: What is **Gluten** and is it bad for you?

You can't help but to hear about Gluten these days, but the main issue to consider is whether or not it's bad for you. Let's take a look. First of all, Gluten is a protein found in many nutritious foods like wheat, barley, and rye. Gluten also shows up in many whole grain foods related to wheat, including bulgur, farro, kamut, spelt, and triticale (a hybrid of wheat and rye). Now, is it good for you or not?

Here's the truth about Gluten: There are a few circumstances where you would be better off eating a Gluten free diet, but other than these, there's no reason to avoid Gluten. The first reason to avoid Gluten is if you have Celiac Disease which affects only about 1% of Americans. Celiac Disease is the condition caused by an abnormal immune response to gluten which can damage the lining of the small intestine. That, in turn, can prevent important nutrients from being absorbed. The second reason would be if you are sensitive to Gluten but even in this case, you most likely would only have to reduce the amount of Gluten you eat rather than completely omit it from your diet.

The truth is, unless you have Celiac Disease or you have sensitivity, avoiding foods that contain Gluten can cause you to miss out on good nutritious foods. Check with your doctor and see what he has to say; then call me and tell me if he agrees with me.

You Ate What???

Are you keeping track of your water? If you are, that's great. But if you aren't, make it a point today to start keeping track and write it in your journal. I also want you to start paying close attention to your total calories and if you are trying to lose weight, start reducing your carbohydrate and fat calories slowly and note all changes in your journal. If you're trying to gain weight, start slowly increasing your carbohydrate calories.

Food Journal

Time of meal 1 - _________

Food eaten- ____

Drink - _______________________

Carbohydrates	**Protein**	**Fat**
Total crab grams -	Total protein grams -	Total fat grams -
Total fiber grams -		
Total sugar grams -		
Total complex grams -		
Total calories of meal -	**cal**	
Total ounces of water with meal -	**ounces**	

Time of meal 2 - _________

Food eaten- ____

Drink - ________________________

Carbohydrates	**Protein**	**Fat**
Total crab grams -	Total protein grams -	Total fat grams -
Total fiber grams -		
Total sugar grams -		
Total complex grams -		

Total calories of meal - **cal**
Total ounces of water with meal - **ounces**

Time of meal 3 - _________

Food eaten- ____

Drink - ________________________

Carbohydrates	**Protein**	**Fat**
Total crab grams -	Total protein grams -	Total fat grams -
Total fiber grams -		
Total sugar grams -		
Total complex grams -		

Total calories of meal - **cal**
Total ounces of water with meal - **ounces**

Time of meal 4 - _________

Food eaten- ____

Drink - ________________________

Carbohydrates	**Protein**	**Fat**
Total crab grams -	Total protein grams -	Total fat grams -
Total fiber grams -		
Total sugar grams -		
Total complex grams -		

Total calories of meal - **cal**
Total ounces of water with meal - **ounces**

Time of meal 5 - _________

Food eaten- ____

Drink - ________________________

Carbohydrates	**Protein**	**Fat**
Total crab grams -	Total protein grams -	Total fat grams -
Total fiber grams -		
Total sugar grams -		
Total complex grams -		

Total calories of meal - cal
Total ounces of water with meal - ounces

Total ounces of water with meals - ounces
Total ounces of water during workout - ounces
Total ounces of water outside meals - ounces
Total ounces of water today - ounces

And The Heart Says…

Tonight after you eat and are sitting down relaxing, take a heart rate and write it down here:

After dinner HR-________ Time taken - ______

Day 1 and 2 are in the books and you know what's coming up tomorrow. That's right; Leg Day! Let's do something a little different tonight before you go to sleep. While you're in bed but right before you go to sleep, visualize how you want your legs to look, and hold that visual for a couple of minutes. That's what I call a head start, or maybe it's a "leg start". See you in the morning!

Round 4 – Day 3

Are your legs rested and ready to go? We're about to find out. There's one sure sign you are recuperating from your workouts: How your legs feel from day to day and how they respond during your leg day workout. Keep an eye on it today and make a few notes in your workout log as to how fresh and lively your legs feel. Okay, let's get it going!

That One Thing

Think about one thing you love to do that you don't do anymore and write it down here.

One thing I love to do that I no longer do is…

Seeing I to Eye

Pick one of your long term career goals and take 3-4 minutes visualizing yourself reaching that goal. Remember to relax and clear your mind before you start visualizing because those negative and worrisome thoughts can take control and wreak havoc on your attempts to picture positive things.

Pre Game

Just like with your "Finishing Strong" post workout section, I'm going to omit it in a few days and only drop it in as a reminder once in a while. I think you've got it by now, right?

Your Workout – See your workout log for today's workout

And the Heart Says…

At any point today after your workout and after you have been sitting for at least 3-4 minutes, take a resting heart rate and record it here.

Resting HR - ______ Time taken - ______

Cleaning Your Plate

Another topic I often hear being discussed around the gym is whether or not every eating plan should have a cheat day built into it. It really depends on how strict you want to be, but if having a day where you eat what you want helps you stay on your eating plan, then I say cheat away. If you do have one cheat day a week, be careful to not let one day turn into two and three days. This is the one of the hazards of having cheat days. Another option for you is to have a few cheat meals across each week instead of having one full cheat day. Personally, I always have at least one cheat meal a week and sometimes two, but that's where it stops for me.

You Ate What???

Are you keeping up with everything? Don't forget to record that water and start taking time to closely look at how many calories of each type of food you are eating. Later on in 12 Rounds, we'll start looking at the ideal ratio between carbs, proteins, and fats.

Food Journal

Time of meal 1 - _________

Food eaten- ____

Drink - ________________________

Carbohydrates	**Protein**	**Fat**
Total crab grams -	Total protein grams -	Total fat grams -
Total fiber grams -		
Total sugar grams -		
Total complex grams -		
Total calories of meal -	**cal**	
Total ounces of water with meal -	**ounces**	

Time of meal 2 - _________

Food eaten- ____

Drink - ________________________

Carbohydrates	**Protein**	**Fat**
Total crab grams -	Total protein grams -	Total fat grams -
Total fiber grams -		
Total sugar grams -		
Total complex grams -		
Total calories of meal -	**cal**	
Total ounces of water with meal -	**ounces**	

Time of meal 3 - _________

Food eaten- ____

Drink - ________________________

Carbohydrates
Total crab grams -
Total fiber grams -
Total sugar grams -
Total complex grams -

Protein
Total protein grams -

Fat
Total fat grams -

Total calories of meal - cal
Total ounces of water with meal - ounces

Time of meal 4 - _________

Food eaten- ____

Drink - ________________________

Carbohydrates
Total crab grams -
Total fiber grams -
Total sugar grams -
Total complex grams -

Protein
Total protein grams -

Fat
Total fat grams -

Total calories of meal - cal
Total ounces of water with meal - ounces

Time of meal 5 - _________

Food eaten- ____

Drink - ________________________

Carbohydrates
Total crab grams -
Total fiber grams -
Total sugar grams -
Total complex grams -

Protein
Total protein grams -

Fat
Total fat grams -

Total calories of meal - cal
Total ounces of water with meal - ounces

Total ounces of water with meals - ounces
Total ounces of water during workout - ounces
Total ounces of water outside meals - ounces
Total ounces of water today - ounces

You had another great day today, and the best thing is, they will keep adding up. Tomorrow is your day off from working out; make sure you keep it that way. I know you may want to work out, but your body and especially your legs need to rest and recuperate. Don't worry; I'll give you plenty to do tomorrow.

Round 4, Day 4

This is going to be a great day for you because you get to take a day off from exercise, but you have other things that will occupy your time. The most important part of 12 Rounds isn't exercise and eating well; it's keeping a positive and healthy mind. That's why I have you set goals, manage your stress, and most importantly; training your mind to think and produce positive outcomes. This is Your Day; now make it a great one!

"Boastful bragging only let's people know how weak you really are. Being confident in your abilities and letting your actions do the talking is where true strength and toughness reside."

Bobby Whisnand

It Happened Just Like This!

In 2007, I decided to get my insurance license and sell long term care insurance for a client of mine. After I got my license my manager asked me to write down daily, weekly, monthly, yearly sales goals. So, that's exactly what I did and after reading them his exact words were, "I like your confidence but I'm going to do you a favor and have you rewrite these. I've never known of anyone come anywhere close to these numbers before and I don't want you to be disappointed." I said, "Give me one month with these goals and if I don't make it, I'll rewrite them." He agreed and off I went.

My first week, I broke the company record and three weeks later, I broke the record for most sales in a month. At the end of the year, I received the agent of the year award from my company and from Mutual of Omaha. I got to spend one week in Atlantis and another week in the Four Seasons Hotel in Las Vegas. Yep, I was feeling awesome! Can't tell you what I did there though.

It's true, I did set my goals a little too high, but deep down I truly believed I could do it. And that, my friend, is where the tire meets the road. The key to reaching your goals and getting where you want to be is first and foremost, believing you can. I'm not talking about thinking you can; that's not enough. You have to dig down deep where your soul lives, get tough, and do what it takes to make it happen. Do you truly believe you can? Show me!

Which Way You Headed?

At this point you have two long term goals on your fitness. Write them both here again and below each one, write how you think you're doing in reaching these goals.

My first long term (12 week) goal on fitness is…

____

In terms of reaching this first long term goal on fitness, I feel I am…

____

My second long term (10 week) goal on my fitness is…

____

In terms of reaching this second long term goal on fitness, I feel I am…

____

Seeing I to Eye

Pick one of your two long term goals on something other than your fitness. Take 3-4 minutes today and visualize yourself reaching that goal. Be as specific as you can and take your time.

Upper Management

It's time to get another point of view about your goals. Contact that person with whom you're sharing your goals and arrange a time to get together. Once you get together, go over all six of your long term goals and discuss how you think you're doing. This is a great motivator; wait and see.

No Workout Today! Enjoy your day off

And the Heart Says…

Take at least one heart rate today whenever you want.

Today I took my heart rate when I was… ____

Day 4 HR - ______ Time taken - ______

Cleaning Your Plate

For one of your meals today, pay very close attention to how much sodium you're getting. In addition, pick one meal and add up how much sodium it is. Just one meal.

You Ate What???

One of the biggest issues in our country and probably the world is consuming too much sodium. When you consume too much sodium your body retains water, adds volume to your blood, and in turn adds pressure to your arteries. This is exactly how too much sodium causes high blood pressure; makes sense doesn't it? For this reason, I want you to journal your sodium intake from just one meal (lunch) a day. We will add days as we go but let's start with one meal a day.

Food Journal

Time of meal 1 - _________

Food eaten- ____

Drink - ________________________

Carbohydrates
Total crab grams -
Total fiber grams -
Total sugar grams -
Total complex grams -

Protein
Total protein grams -

Fat
Total fat grams -

Total calories of meal - cal
Total ounces of water with meal - ounces

Time of meal 2 - _________

Food eaten- ____

Drink - ________________________

Carbohydrates
Total crab grams -
Total fiber grams -
Total sugar grams -
Total complex grams -

Protein
Total protein grams -

Fat
Total fat grams -

Total calories of meal - **cal**
Total ounces of water with meal - **ounces**

Time of meal 3 (Lunch) - _________

Food eaten- ____

Drink - ________________________

Carbohydrates
Total crab grams -
Total fiber grams -
Total sugar grams -
Total complex grams -

Protein
Total protein grams -

Fat
Total fat grams -

Total calories of meal - **cal**
Total ounces of water with meal - **ounces**
Total sodium of meal - **mgs**

Time of meal 4 - _________

Food eaten- ____

Drink - ________________________

Carbohydrates
Total crab grams -
Total fiber grams -
Total sugar grams -
Total complex grams -

Protein
Total protein grams -

Fat
Total fat grams -

Total calories of meal - **cal**
Total ounces of water with meal - **ounces**

Time of meal 5 - _________

Food eaten- ____

Drink - ________________________

Carbohydrates	**Protein**	**Fat**
Total crab grams -	Total protein grams -	Total fat grams -
Total fiber grams -		
Total sugar grams -		
Total complex grams -		

Total calories of meal - cal
Total ounces of water with meal - ounces

Total ounces of water with meals - ounces
Total ounces of water outside meals - ounces
Total ounces of water today - ounces

Day 4 is almost over but there's one more thing I want you to think about. If you counted the hours from the time you finished dinner and the time you eat breakfast in the morning, you're going to see about 10-12 hours go by without eating. That's a very long time to be without food; even though you were mostly sleeping. One of the absolute best things you can do to get your body and brain started on the right track is to always eat a good clean breakfast. No Pop Tarts either. I'll see you tomorrow champ.

Round 4 - Day 5

Oh yes! It's Day 5 and you know what that means. It's back and biceps day so get that body and brain going so we can get to it. Don't forget to log your breakfast before you get too far behind and put a smile on that face while you're at it.

That One Thing

On Day 3 of this week, I asked you to write down one thing you love to do that you don't do anymore. Write it down again here along with one thing you can do today that will help you to start doing it again.

The one thing I love to do that I don't do anymore is…

____

The one thing that I can do TODAY that will help me to start doing it again is…

____

Seeing I to Eye

Here's a new one for you: Take 4-5 minutes and visualize helping someone else reach one of the two fitness goals you have. You're a great teacher, you just don't know it.

Your Workout – See your workout log for today's workout

And the Heart Says…

Some time tonight after dinner and when you have been relaxing for about an hour, take and record a heart rate.

Evening resting HR ______ Time taken - ______

Cleaning Your Plate

At the end of the day yesterday, I talked about how long your body has been without food overnight. The exact same thing goes for water and one of the best ways to get everything about your body and mind going in the right direction is to drink 10-12 ounces of water as soon as you get up in the morning. Your body will love you for it.

You Ate What???

How much sodium are you consuming during lunch? You're measuring this right? I hope so because coming up very soon, we're going to start making healthy changes to your awesome food journal, and I want this to be one of them. Start paying close attention to how much fat your getting in your daily eating and start reducing it if it's adding up to a lot of calories.

Food Journal

Time of meal 1 - _________

Food eaten- ____

Drink - ________________________

Carbohydrates
Total crab grams -
Total fiber grams -
Total sugar grams -
Total complex grams -

Protein
Total protein grams -

Fat
Total fat grams -

Total calories of meal - cal
Total ounces of water with meal - ounces

Time of meal 2 - _________

Food eaten- ____

Drink - ________________________

Carbohydrates
Total crab grams -
Total fiber grams -
Total sugar grams -
Total complex grams -

Protein
Total protein grams -

Fat
Total fat grams -

Total calories of meal - cal
Total ounces of water with meal - ounces

Time of meal 3 (Lunch) - _________

Food eaten- ____

Drink - ________________________

Carbohydrates	**Protein**	**Fat**
Total crab grams -	Total protein grams -	Total fat grams -
Total fiber grams -		
Total sugar grams -		
Total complex grams -		

Total calories of meal - cal
Total ounces of water with meal - ounces
Total sodium of meal - mgs

Time of meal 4 - _________

Food eaten- ____

Drink - ________________________

Carbohydrates	**Protein**	**Fat**
Total crab grams -	Total protein grams -	Total fat grams -
Total fiber grams -		
Total sugar grams -		
Total complex grams -		

Total calories of meal - cal
Total ounces of water with meal - ounces

Time of meal 5 - _________

Food eaten- ____

Drink - ________________________

Carbohydrates	**Protein**	**Fat**
Total crab grams -	Total protein grams -	Total fat grams -
Total fiber grams -		
Total sugar grams -		
Total complex grams -		

Total calories of meal - cal
Total ounces of water with meal - ounces

Total ounces of water with meals - ounces
Total ounces of water during workout - ounces
Total ounces of water outside meals - ounces
Total ounces of water today - ounces

How are those guns feeling? Did you work them out good today? That unilateral high rep reverse workout puts a pretty serious burn on those biceps doesn't it? Now it's time to recuperate those muscles and get ready for tomorrow because it's your core's turn to burn. Sleep tight and dream big!

Round 4 - Day 6

And just like that, there was Day 6. What's up today? Did you get enough sleep? Oh, and did you drink 10-12 ounces of water as soon as you got up and eat a good clean breakfast? These two things make some of the biggest impacts on how fit you become so don't skip them. Let's go get this Day 6!

Which Way You Headed?

You have two long term goals about your career at this point. Write them in the spaces below and underneath each goal, write down how you think you're doing to this point.

My first long term (12 week) goal about my career is -

____

In terms of reaching this first long term goal about my career, I feel I am…

____

My second long term (10 week) goal about my career is…

____

In terms of reaching this second long term goal about my career, I feel I am…

____

Upper Management

On Day 6 of Round 3, you rewrote the list of things you need to get done and off your mind. Write it again on a piece of paper and put it where you can see it every day like on your refrigerator, on your desk, or anywhere you'll see it easily. Now you were supposed to check a few things off that list by now but if you haven't, you better catch up because by the end of 12 Rounds, we're going to get all of them done and off that list.

Seeing I to Eye

Take 4-5 minutes today and visualize the abdominals you want. This is a tough one but you can do it. Six pack on the way. As always, clear your mind and relax before you start your visualization.

Your Workout – See your workout log for today's workout.

And the Heart Says…

You took a lot of heart rates today but that's a good thing. I want you to take one more so we can see how your heart is recovering from that awesome workout today. At some point this evening when you are relaxed, take another heart rate and record it here.

Post workout HR ______ Time taken - ______

Cleaning Your Plate

We are getting very close to the point where you are going to start evaluating your food journal. It's really easy to do and we will start slowly but it's the bread and butter of making good changes in your eating. Get it? Bread and butter? Keep this food journal going and no matter what or when you eat and drink, write EVERYTHING down so we can start cleaning it up.

You Ate What???

Food Journal

Time of meal 1 - _________

Food eaten- ____

Drink - ________________________

Carbohydrates	**Protein**	**Fat**
Total crab grams -	Total protein grams -	Total fat grams -
Total fiber grams -		
Total sugar grams -		
Total complex grams -		

Total calories of meal - **cal**
Total ounces of water with meal - **ounces**

Time of meal 2 - _________

Food eaten- ____

Drink - ________________________

Carbohydrates	**Protein**	**Fat**
Total crab grams -	Total protein grams -	Total fat grams -
Total fiber grams -		
Total sugar grams -		
Total complex grams -		

Total calories of meal - **cal**
Total ounces of water with meal - **ounces**

Time of meal 3 (Lunch) - _________

Food eaten- ____

Drink - ________________________

Carbohydrates	**Protein**	**Fat**
Total crab grams -	Total protein grams -	Total fat grams -
Total fiber grams -		
Total sugar grams -		
Total complex grams -		

Total calories of meal - **cal**
Total ounces of water with meal - **ounces**
Total sodium of meal - **mgs**

Time of meal 4 - ________

Food eaten- ____

Drink - _____________________

Carbohydrates	**Protein**	**Fat**
Total crab grams -	Total protein grams -	Total fat grams -
Total fiber grams -		
Total sugar grams -		
Total complex grams -		
Total calories of meal - **cal**		
Total ounces of water with meal - **ounces**		

Time of meal 5 - ________

Food eaten- ____

Drink - _____________________

Carbohydrates	**Protein**	**Fat**
Total crab grams -	Total protein grams -	Total fat grams -
Total fiber grams -		
Total sugar grams -		
Total complex grams -		
Total calories of meal - **cal**		
Total ounces of water with meal - **ounces**		

Total ounces of water with meals - **ounces**
Total ounces of water during workout - **ounces**
Total ounces of water outside meals - **ounces**
Total ounces of water today - **ounces**

This about does it for Round 4. As usual, tomorrow is your day off from 12 Rounds but just in case you want to take a heart rate or journal your food, I've got places for you to do that. Another outstanding day for you, and now it's time to relax, eat some good food, go out with some friends, and enjoy your life. I'll see you soon.

Round 4 - Day 7

Good morning! How do you feel from yesterday's core and cardio circuit? We added some time to that workout and you may be feeling it today so take it easy and don't exercise today. If you want, you can look back over what you've done to this point or you can look at the appendix in the back and take a look at how you're workout is going to change starting tomorrow; it's another good one with a lot of changes, but you can handle it. Enjoy your day, and I'll see you tomorrow for the start of Round 5!

Day 7 HR ______ **Time taken -** ______

Food Journal

Time of meal 1 - _________

Food eaten- ____

Drink - ________________________

Carbohydrates	**Protein**	**Fat**
Total crab grams -	Total protein grams -	Total fat grams -
Total fiber grams -		
Total sugar grams -		
Total complex grams -		
Total calories of meal -	**cal**	
Total ounces of water with meal -	**ounces**	

Time of meal 2 - _________

Food eaten- ____

Drink - ________________________

Carbohydrates	**Protein**	**Fat**
Total crab grams -	Total protein grams -	Total fat grams -
Total fiber grams -		
Total sugar grams -		
Total complex grams -		
Total calories of meal -	**cal**	
Total ounces of water with meal -	**ounces**	

Time of meal 3 (Lunch) - _________

Food eaten- ____

Drink - ________________________

Carbohydrates	**Protein**	**Fat**
Total crab grams -	Total protein grams -	Total fat grams -
Total fiber grams -		
Total sugar grams -		
Total complex grams -		
Total calories of meal -	**cal**	
Total ounces of water with meal -	**ounces**	
Total sodium of meal -	**mgs**	

Time of meal 4 - _________

Food eaten- ____

Drink - ________________________

Carbohydrates	**Protein**	**Fat**
Total crab grams -	Total protein grams -	Total fat grams -
Total fiber grams -		
Total sugar grams -		
Total complex grams -		

Total calories of meal - **cal**
Total ounces of water with meal - **ounces**

Time of meal 5 - _________

Food eaten- ____

Drink - ________________________

Carbohydrates	**Protein**	**Fat**
Total crab grams -	Total protein grams -	Total fat grams -
Total fiber grams -		
Total sugar grams -		
Total complex grams -		

Total calories of meal - **cal**
Total ounces of water with meal - **ounces**

Total ounces of water with meals - **ounces**
Total ounces of water outside meals - **ounces**
Total ounces of water today - **ounces**

Round 5 – It's All Heart

Day 1

At this point, you've made some really big changes in your life and these changes are going to start showing up in big ways. But the biggest change of all for you is happening right now in your heart; the most important muscle in your entire body. Your hear t is affected in a lot more ways than how you exercise and eat; it's affected just as much by how you think. That's a big reason why I have you take heart rates during the days when you're *not* exercising, why I give you ways to manage your stress, and why I have you visualize positive things every day. Just like I always say, "Considering every little thing in your life, without a doubt, **It's All Heart**".

Bring on Round 5!

"When it comes down to that very moment when you're fighting, loving, weeping, caring, or living, there's only one thing and one thing only that it begins and ends with every single time...your heart."

Bobby Whisnand

It Happened Just Like This!

It was Valentine's Day and I was speaking on behalf of the American Heart Association in Dallas. After I was introduced, I looked out at everyone, and said, "I want every single one of you to think about the longest relationship you have ever had. Now, I can tell every single one of you what your longest relationship has been and exactly how long it is by simply knowing your age. Do I have a volunteer?" A gentleman about half way back in the audience raised his hand and I asked how old he was. He said he was 52 years old. I then said, "The longest relationship you have ever had is 52 years and nine months and that relationship, my friend, is with your heart." The entire audience broke out into applause and the rest of the presentation was awesome!

Before you were even born, your heart accepted the unconditional responsibility of taking care of you for the rest of your life, no matter how you treat it. Don't you think you should return the favor?

That One Thing

Today when you get into your vehicle, take a look at the odometer and see what your mileage is and write it down here:

The mileage on my vehicle is __________miles.

How many miles are on your other vehicle, the one on two legs? And yes, you do have an odometer on your heart and the rest of your body; you just have to know how to read it.

Seeing I to Eye

Think of one thing you're good at doing and take a few minutes today visualizing yourself doing that one thing. Also, write that one thing down here, and don't hold back. It's Your 12 Rounds, right?

That one thing I'm good at doing is...

____

Your Workout – See your workout log for today's workout.

And the Heart Says…

Tonight when you are lying in bed and before you go to sleep, take one more heart rate and write it down here.

Pre Sleep HR - ______ Time taken - ______

Cleaning Your Plate

So far we have covered quite a few topics on nutrition, but if you want more information on any topics we have covered or other topics, here are two great resources you can use. These are the same resources I use when I research something on nutrition.

- **American Heart Association – www.heart.org**
- **The Mayo Clinic – www.mayoclinic.org**

You Ate What???

Okay, I've added something else for you to do with your food journal. Don't get mad at me. For two of your meals today, place a check mark beside the food you ate that was a good choice, and for the food you ate that was not a good choice, write down what would have been better to eat. In a few weeks, we'll address the exact amounts of each food you should be eating.

Food Journal

Time of meal 1 - _________

Food eaten- ____

Drink - ________________________

Carbohydrates	**Protein**	**Fat**
Total crab grams -	Total protein grams -	Total fat grams -
Total fiber grams -		
Total sugar grams -		
Total complex grams -		

Total calories of meal - cal
Total ounces of water with meal - ounces

Time of meal 2 - _________

Food eaten- ____

Drink - ________________________

Carbohydrates	**Protein**	**Fat**
Total crab grams -	Total protein grams -	Total fat grams -
Total fiber grams -		
Total sugar grams -		
Total complex grams -		

Total calories of meal - **cal**

Total ounces of water with meal - **ounces**

Time of meal 3 (Lunch) - _________

Food eaten- ____

Drink - ________________________

Carbohydrates	**Protein**	**Fat**
Total crab grams -	Total protein grams -	Total fat grams -
Total fiber grams -		
Total sugar grams -		
Total complex grams -		

Total calories of meal - **cal**

Total ounces of water with meal - **ounces**

Total sodium of meal - **mgs**

Time of meal 4 - _________

Food eaten- ____

Drink - ________________________

Carbohydrates	**Protein**	**Fat**
Total crab grams -	Total protein grams -	Total fat grams -
Total fiber grams -		
Total sugar grams -		
Total complex grams -		

Total calories of meal - **cal**

Total ounces of water with meal - **ounces**

Time of meal 5 - _________

Food eaten- ____

Drink - ________________________

Carbohydrates	**Protein**	**Fat**
Total crab grams -	Total protein grams -	Total fat grams -
Total fiber grams -		
Total sugar grams -		
Total complex grams -		

Total calories of meal - **cal**

Total ounces of water with meal - **ounces**

Total ounces of water with meals - ounces
Total ounces of water during workout - ounces
Total ounces of water outside meals - ounces
Total ounces of water today - ounces

That's a great start to Round 5 my friend! With each day you complete, you're paving the way to success. And the best part about all of it; you're doing it on your terms. Keep at it, stay tough, and stick tight to this program and everything will fall into place. You'll see.

Round 5, Day 2

I got plenty of sleep last night, did you? How about that heart rate you took before you went to bed; was it pretty low? Speaking of your heart, what's it doing right now? Let's take a quick heart rate and write it down before we really get going today.

Morning HR - ______ Time taken - ________

Which Way You Headed?

So far you have two goals that are about something other than fitness. Last week you wrote down how you felt you were doing with both goals and you reviewed them with a friend. Today, I want you to closely evaluate these two goals and adjust them as needed.

My first long term (12 week) goal about something other than my fitness is...

____

What adjustments do I need with this first goal if any?

____

My second long term (10 week) goal about something other than my fitness is...

____

What adjustments do I need with this second goal if any?

____

Seeing I to Eye

Today I want you to think about another talent you wish you had like being able to play professional sports, singing, playing an instrument, public speaking, being a dancing machine, etc. Once you have it, take 3-4 minutes and visualize yourself using this talent but this time, add a crowd or audience, put your favorite music with it, and be as specific as you can by seeing actual faces of the people around you.

The talent I wish I had but the one I can definitely see myself doing in a crowd is...

____

Upper Management

Almost all of us worry somewhat about our financial future. Think of one thing you can start doing this week to save money and write it down.

One thing I can start doing this week to help me save money for my future is…

____

Your Workout – See your workout log for today's workout.

Cleaning Your Plate

I know you hear a lot about the importance of getting enough protein to support your muscles, bones, and hormone production, but is protein a good source of energy? This is actually a two part answer. Protein can be a source of energy for your body but the process to break it down to be used as an energy source takes a lot longer than it does for carbohydrates and fats. The fact is, your body has other uses for protein that are essential like muscle, bone, and hormone support rather than to be used as an energy source. So, protein can be a source of energy for you, but it's not the best source and can rob your body of other important processes. Your best sources of energy are carbohydrates, ingested fat, and body fat. Is that easy enough? Good!

You Ate What???

For two of your meals today, place a check mark beside the food you ate that was a good choice, and for the food you ate that was not a good choice, write down what would have been better to eat. Keep an eye on the amount of calorie differences between your carbs, proteins, and fats.

Food Journal

Time of meal 1 - _________

Food eaten- ____

Drink - ________________________

Carbohydrates	**Protein**	**Fat**
Total crab grams -	Total protein grams -	Total fat grams -
Total fiber grams -		
Total sugar grams -		
Total complex grams -		
Total calories of meal -	**cal**	
Total ounces of water with meal -	**ounces**	

Time of meal 2 - _________

Food eaten- ____

Drink - ________________________

Carbohydrates	**Protein**	**Fat**
Total crab grams -	Total protein grams -	Total fat grams -
Total fiber grams -		
Total sugar grams -		
Total complex grams -		
Total calories of meal -	**cal**	
Total ounces of water with meal -	**ounces**	

Time of meal 3 (Lunch) - ________

Food eaten- ____

Drink - ________________________

Carbohydrates	**Protein**	**Fat**
Total crab grams -	Total protein grams -	Total fat grams -
Total fiber grams -		
Total sugar grams -		
Total complex grams -		
Total calories of meal -	**cal**	
Total ounces of water with meal -	**ounces**	
Total sodium of meal -	**mgs**	

Time of meal 4 - ________

Food eaten- ____

Drink - ________________________

Carbohydrates	**Protein**	**Fat**
Total crab grams -	Total protein grams -	Total fat grams -
Total fiber grams -		
Total sugar grams -		
Total complex grams -		
Total calories of meal -	**cal**	
Total ounces of water with meal -	**ounces**	

Time of meal 5 - ________

Food eaten- ____

Drink - ________________________

Carbohydrates	**Protein**	**Fat**
Total crab grams -	Total protein grams -	Total fat grams -
Total fiber grams -		
Total sugar grams -		
Total complex grams -		
Total calories of meal -	**cal**	
Total ounces of water with meal -	**ounces**	

Total ounces of water with meals - ounces
Total ounces of water during workout - ounces
Total ounces of water outside meals - ounces
Total ounces of water today - ounces

And The Heart Says…

Tonight after you eat and are sitting down relaxing, take a heart rate and write it down here:

After dinner HR-________ Time taken - _______

Here we are at the end of another day; Great Job! One thing you can start doing each night is looking at the appendix in the back and reviewing your workout coming up the next day. Even though these are my workout logs, they will help you get a close gauge on how much weight you're going to need. So take a look and if you want; you can even write the weights in your workout log that you think you'll be using for your exercises coming up the next day. This will save a lot of time and keep you on track, especially on those "light" days. Sleep tight; I'll see you tomorrow for LEG DAY!

Round 5 – Day 3

What are we doing today? Is it back and biceps day? Is it Abs day? NOPE! It's good old LEG DAY! Doing a leg workout burns a lot of calories so make sure you are eating good food within 30 minutes after your workout and don't forget to STRETCH. Let's kick it off!

That One Thing

We know that exercising and eating right helps you have a healthy heart, but what else can you do to help your heart help you?
One thing I can do today to help my heart other than exercise and eating right is…

____

Seeing I to Eye

You've taken a ton of heart rates with 12 Rounds which is a very important thing to do. Today, let's actually visualize your heart beating. Find your heart rate and as you're feeling your heart beat, visualize your actual heart beating in your chest. That my friend is the purest form of life, right there just to the left of the center of your chest. Take care of it; you're all its got.

Your Workout – See your workout log for today's workout

And the Heart Says…

At any point today after your workout and after you have been sitting for at least 3-4 minutes, take a resting heart rate and record it here.

Resting HR - ______ Time Taken - ________

Cleaning Your Plate

One thing I love about parties is all the great FOOD! And the best part is you don't have to make it or clean up after you're done unless you're the one throwing it. Either way, this is where it's very easy to get way off course from your normal eating plan. Are you shaking your head? You should definitely enjoy yourself at these parties but if you want to stay as close to your diet as possible, do this one thing right before you go: EAT! That's right; have a good clean meal right before you go to the party and this will help you not to eat so much once you're there. It's definitely no guarantee, but it does help, unless you're me. Me at a party with good food = cookie monster, big time!

You Ate What???

When you're marking your two meals for good and bad choices today, try marking two different meals than the ones you marked the first two days this week. Pretty soon, we will be marking all meals like this; I know you're excited about that aren't you?

Food Journal

Time of meal 1 - _________

Food eaten- ____

Drink - ________________________

Carbohydrates	**Protein**	**Fat**
Total crab grams -	Total protein grams -	Total fat grams -
Total fiber grams -		
Total sugar grams -		
Total complex grams -		
Total calories of meal -	**cal**	
Total ounces of water with meal -	**ounces**	

Time of meal 2 - _________

Food eaten- ____

Drink - ________________________

Carbohydrates	**Protein**	**Fat**
Total crab grams -	Total protein grams -	Total fat grams -
Total fiber grams -		
Total sugar grams -		
Total complex grams -		
Total calories of meal -	**cal**	
Total ounces of water with meal -	**ounces**	

Time of meal 3 (Lunch) - _________

Food eaten- ____

Drink - ________________________

Carbohydrates	**Protein**	**Fat**
Total crab grams -	Total protein grams -	Total fat grams -
Total fiber grams -		
Total sugar grams -		
Total complex grams -		
Total calories of meal -	**cal**	
Total ounces of water with meal -	**ounces**	

Time of meal 4 - _________

Food eaten- ____

Drink - ________________________

Carbohydrates	**Protein**	**Fat**
Total crab grams -	Total protein grams -	Total fat grams -
Total fiber grams -		
Total sugar grams -		
Total complex grams -		
Total calories of meal -	**cal**	
Total ounces of water with meal -	**ounces**	

Time of meal 5 - _________

Food eaten- ____

Drink - ________________________

Carbohydrates	**Protein**	**Fat**
Total crab grams -	Total protein grams -	Total fat grams -
Total fiber grams -		
Total sugar grams -		
Total complex grams -		
Total calories of meal -	**cal**	
Total ounces of water with meal -	**ounces**	

Total ounces of water with meals - **ounces**
Total ounces of water during workout - **ounces**
Total ounces of water outside meals - **ounces**
Total ounces of water today - **ounces**

I know I have said this several times at the end of your day, but the importance of sleep cannot be overlooked. If you are getting 7-8 hours of good quality sleep, you're in a great place. If you are someone who has trouble falling asleep and/or getting good quality sleep, take a look at the link below for a list of ways to help you sleep from the Mayo Clinic. For me, it's a cold dark room where I can't hear anything; that's my way to long quality sleeping. I'll see you tomorrow!

Better Sleep - *http://www.mayoclinic.org/healthy-lifestyle/adult-health/in-depth/sleep/art-20048379*

Round 5, Day 4

"The heart: A shelter for a thousand feelings, fears, loves, pains, and joys, and it always has room for more."
Bobby Whisnand

It Happened Just Like This!

Your Heart: The muscle that determines how good you're going to be on any day, week, month, or year of your life. The thing is; your heart can very easily turn into an "out of sight out of mind" thing which often leads to it being taken for granted. If you want to have the best heart you can possibly have, you have to put it in the front of your mind every single day and do the things it needs for both of you to be healthy and happy. Heart disease is a very big problem in our country, and just so you'll know just how big and common of a problem it is, I'm going to give you these statistics from the **Centers for Disease Control and Prevention.**

- About 610,000 people die of heart disease in the United States every year–that's 1 in every 4 deaths.
- Heart disease is the leading cause of death for both men and women.
- Coronary heart disease is the most common type of heart disease, killing over 370,000 people annually.
- Every year about 735,000 Americans have a heart attack. Of these, 525,000 are a first heart attack and 210,000 happen in people who have already had a heart attack.

You've only got one; take care of it!

Which Way You Headed?

So far you have two goals that are about your fitness. Last week you wrote down how you felt you were doing with both goals and you reviewed them with a friend. Today, I want you to closely evaluate these two goals and adjust them as needed.

My first long term (12 week) goal about my fitness is...

____

What adjustments do I need with this first goal if any?

____

My second long term (10 week) goal about my fitness is...

____

What adjustments do I need with this second goal if any?

____

Seeing I to Eye

Get to that quiet place where there are no distractions, and once you're there, think about an event in your life where you were very proud of yourself. Take 4-5 minutes and enjoy this memory and then write that proud memory down here:

The event in my life when I was very proud of myself was…

____

Upper Management

One of the best ways to manage stress is to make a short escape. Think about something that's fun for you to do that you can afford and make a plan to do it. You can do things like go to a movie, shopping, take a long ride, go to a nice park, visit a museum or art gallery, or anything you like to do that will give you a break from thinking about stressful things.

No Workout Today! Enjoy your day off

And the Heart Says…

Take at least one heart rate today whenever you want. Just make sure you write down when and under what circumstances you took it.

Today I took my heart rate when I was… ____

Day 4 HR - ______ Time Taken - ________

Cleaning Your Plate

"No Sugar Added"

How many times have you seen this on a food or drink label? I see it all the time and the truth is it doesn't mean that much at all. This is a great way for food companies to get your attention and make you think it's a low sugar food or drink when in fact, it more than likely isn't. Food companies can put that on any label as long as they don't actually add sugar to the food or drink item. It absolutely does not mean that a certain food or drink is low in sugar.

Read those labels carefully; you have enough experience by now.

You Ate What???

Keep journaling your food as before, but tomorrow we're going to add a few more meals for you to evaluate, as well as keeping track of your sodium for all meals. I know; just what you were wanting to hear, right?

Food Journal

Time of meal 1 - _________

Food eaten- ____

Drink - ________________________

Carbohydrates	**Protein**	**Fat**
Total crab grams -	Total protein grams -	Total fat grams -
Total fiber grams -		
Total sugar grams -		
Total complex grams -		

Total calories of meal - cal
Total ounces of water with meal - ounces

Time of meal 2 - _________

Food eaten- ____

Drink - ________________________

Carbohydrates	**Protein**	**Fat**
Total crab grams -	Total protein grams -	Total fat grams -
Total fiber grams -		
Total sugar grams -		
Total complex grams -		

Total calories of meal - cal
Total ounces of water with meal - ounces

Time of meal 3 (Lunch) - _________

Food eaten- ____

Drink - ________________________

Carbohydrates	**Protein**	**Fat**
Total crab grams -	Total protein grams -	Total fat grams -
Total fiber grams -		
Total sugar grams -		
Total complex grams -		

Total calories of meal - cal
Total ounces of water with meal - ounces
Total sodium of meal - mgs

Time of meal 4 - _________

Food eaten- ____

Drink - ________________________

Carbohydrates	**Protein**	**Fat**
Total crab grams -	Total protein grams -	Total fat grams -
Total fiber grams -		
Total sugar grams -		
Total complex grams -		

Total calories of meal - cal
Total ounces of water with meal - ounces

Time of meal 5 - _________

Food eaten- ____

Drink - ________________________

Carbohydrates
Total crab grams -
Total fiber grams -
Total sugar grams -
Total complex grams -

Protein
Total protein grams -

Fat
Total fat grams -

Total calories of meal - cal
Total ounces of water with meal - ounces

Total ounces of water with meals - ounces
Total ounces of water during workout - ounces
Total ounces of water outside meals - ounces
Total ounces of water today - ounces

You are right smack dab in the middle of 12 Rounds; you've got a food journal that's looking awesome, and your body, mind, and heart are getting healthier by the day. How are you feeling at this point? However it is, it's only going to get better. One thing I want to put in your mind is about your food journal. Starting tomorrow, we're going to start tracking your sodium intake for all meals, and on Day 6, we're going to add another meal to evaluate. It does take some time, but it's no big deal for a champion like you. Go rest up, put that mind in a positive place, and I'll go get the gym ready for your "out of this world" bike and bicep workout tomorrow.

Round 5 - Day 5

Are you ready for another great Day 5? Although Leg Day is my favorite workout day, I do love a good back and bicep workout. How about you? What is your favorite workout day? What do you think about those reverse workouts? They are definitely different but they do have their place. Let's go do this!

That One Thing

Ask yourself this one question: Do you know your blood pressure and cholesterol numbers? These are what are known as the "silent killers" because they typically have so symptoms. The one thing I want you to do today is think about your numbers and if you don't know them, make an appointment with your doctor to get them checked. I'm counting on you. Did you get that one?

Seeing I to Eye

Think back to when you made someone feel good about themselves. Once you have it, take 4-5 minutes today visualizing that person feeling great, as well as how it made you feel. Doing or saying something to make someone's day better or to make someone feel better about themselves is priceless, and it takes so little effort. This is what takes up more room in my heart than anything else.

Your Workout – See your workout log for today's workout

And the Heart Says…

Some time tonight after dinner and when you have been relaxing for about an hour, take and record a heart rate.

Evening resting HR ______ Time taken ______

Cleaning Your Plate

Have you ever wondered about the difference between table salt and sea salt?

I hear a lot of people talk about the fact that they use sea salt because it's healthier than table salt when in fact, there is very little difference. The most notable differences between sea salt and table salt are in their taste, texture and processing.

Sea salt is produced through evaporation of ocean water or water from saltwater lakes, usually with little processing. Table salt is typically mined from underground salt deposits. Table salt is more heavily processed to eliminate minerals and usually contains an additive to prevent clumping. Most table salt also has added iodine, an essential nutrient that helps maintain a healthy thyroid.

Sea salt and table salt have the same basic nutritional value, despite the fact that sea salt is often promoted as being healthier. Sea salt and table salt contain comparable amounts of sodium by weight. There you go, so the next time somebody brings up this topic, you'll know exactly what to say.

You Ate What???

Okay, here's the one change I want you to make to your food journal from here on out: Start journaling how much sodium you're getting with each meal instead of just one meal a day. Just take a little extra time and read those labels and you'll do fine.

Food Journal

Time of meal 1 - ________

Food eaten- ____

Drink - ______________________

Carbohydrates	**Protein**	**Fat**
Total crab grams -	Total protein grams -	Total fat grams -
Total fiber grams -		
Total sugar grams -		
Total complex grams -		
Total calories of meal -	**cal**	
Total ounces of water with meal -	**ounces**	
Total sodium of meal -	**mgs**	

Time of meal 2 - ________

Food eaten- ____

Drink - ______________________

Carbohydrates | **Protein** | **Fat**
Total crab grams - | Total protein grams - | Total fat grams -
Total fiber grams -
Total sugar grams -
Total complex grams -
Total calories of meal - cal
Total ounces of water with meal - ounces
Total sodium of meal - mgs

Time of meal 3 (Lunch) - _________

Food eaten- ____

Drink - ________________________

Carbohydrates | **Protein** | **Fat**
Total crab grams - | Total protein grams - | Total fat grams -
Total fiber grams -
Total sugar grams -
Total complex grams -
Total calories of meal - cal
Total ounces of water with meal - ounces
Total sodium of meal - mgs

Time of meal 4 - _________

Food eaten- ____

Drink - ________________________

Carbohydrates | **Protein** | **Fat**
Total crab grams - | Total protein grams - | Total fat grams -
Total fiber grams -
Total sugar grams -
Total complex grams -
Total calories of meal - cal
Total ounces of water with meal - ounces
Total sodium of meal - mgs

Time of meal 5 - _________

Food eaten- ____

Drink - ________________________

Carbohydrates	**Protein**	**Fat**
Total crab grams -	Total protein grams -	Total fat grams -
Total fiber grams -		
Total sugar grams -		
Total complex grams -		

Total calories of meal - **cal**
Total ounces of water with meal - **ounces**
Total sodium of meal - **mgs**

Total ounces of water with meals - **ounces**
Total ounces of water during workout - **ounces**
Total ounces of water outside meals - **ounces**
Total ounces of water today - **ounces**
Total sodium today - **mgs**

12 Rounds is great isn't it? I think the best things about it is how often it changes, how you get to learn and clear up misconceptions about nutrition, and how you learn to improve all parts of your life. There are a lot of things that can help you have a better life; sometimes you just have to be reminded of them, and that's why I'm here. Keep your head up, keep the arrow pointing forward, and be very proud of yourself; you're moving toward a better life with every single day that goes by. Go get some good food and some good sleep; I'll be waiting and ready for you to knock Day 6 right off its feet.

Round 5 - Day 6

Okay sleepy head, I've been up for hours waiting on you. Make sure you go drink that glass of water before you do anything else and get some good clean food in you because today's workout is going to be a tough one. Let me know when you're ready to roll. Look at that; a little rhyme.

Which Way You Headed?

So far you have two goals that are about your career. Last week you wrote down how you felt you were doing with both goals and you reviewed them with a friend. Today, I want you to closely evaluate these two goals and adjust them as needed.

My first long term (12 week) goal about my career is…

____

What adjustments do I need with this first goal if any?

____

My second long term (10 week) goal about my career is…

____

What adjustments do I need with this second goal if any?

____

Upper Management

For today, I want you to take a close look at just how far you've come. Write down three things you are doing better today than you were before starting this program.

The first thing I've improved in my life with 12 Rounds is...

____

The second thing I've improved in my life with 12 Rounds is...

____

The third thing I've improved in my life with 12 Rounds is...

____

Seeing I to Eye

It's your choice today. Take some time to be by yourself and visualize anything you want. Maybe it's a trip you took, being with your family during the holidays, your first car, or anything that makes you feel good. Make it like you're really there all over again; you know how!

Your Workout – See your workout log for today's workout.

And the Heart Says…

At some point this evening when you are relaxed, take another heart rate and record it here.

Post workout evening HR ______ Time taken __________

Cleaning Your Plate

There is a lot of talk about the importance of taking Omega oils, but what exactly are they and why are they good for you to take?

Monounsaturated and polyunsaturated fats are known by another name: omegas. There are three types of omega fatty acids: omega-3, omega-6 and omega-9. Omega-3 and omega-6 fatty acids are two types of polyunsaturated fat. They are considered essential fatty acids because the body cannot manufacture them. Omega-9 fatty acids are from a family of monounsaturated fats that also are beneficial when obtained in food. Omega-9 Canola and Sunflower Oils are uniquely high in omega-9 (monounsaturated) fatty acid.

All omega fatty acids play specific roles in overall health. These good fats can have health benefits, including:

- Prevent coronary heart disease
- Prevent stroke
- Prevent diabetes
- Promote healthy nerve activity
- Improve vitamin absorption

- Maintain a healthy immune system
- Promote cell development

Great sources of Omega 3 oils are Flax seeds, walnuts, soybeans, navy beans, kidney beans, fish, avocado, and some dark green leafy vegetables.

Great sources of Omega 6 oils are flax seeds, pumpkin seeds, and grapeseed oil.

Great sources of Omega 9 oils are nuts, avocados, and olive oil.

If you want to learn more about the Omega oils and how they benefit your body, use the following link and resource to learn all you need to know.

http://www.webmd.com/vitamins-and-supplements/lifestyle-guide-11/supplement-guide-omega-3-fatty-acids

You Ate What???

As you're journaling your meals, be sure you're keeping track of your sodium intakes for all meals and that you're marking two meals a day for both good and bad choices. You're doing great; keep it up!

Food Journal

Time of meal 1 - ________

Food eaten- ____

Drink - ________________________

Carbohydrates	**Protein**	**Fat**
Total crab grams -	Total protein grams -	Total fat grams -
Total fiber grams -		
Total sugar grams -		
Total complex grams -		

Total calories of meal - **cal**
Total ounces of water with meal - **ounces**
Total sodium of meal - **mgs**

Time of meal 2 - ________

Food eaten- ____

Drink - ________________________

Carbohydrates	**Protein**	**Fat**
Total crab grams -	Total protein grams -	Total fat grams -
Total fiber grams -		
Total sugar grams -		
Total complex grams -		

Total calories of meal - **cal**
Total ounces of water with meal - **ounces**
Total sodium of meal - **mgs**

Time of meal 3 (Lunch) - ________

Food eaten- ____

Drink - ________________________

Carbohydrates	**Protein**	**Fat**
Total crab grams -	Total protein grams -	Total fat grams -
Total fiber grams -		
Total sugar grams -		
Total complex grams -		
Total calories of meal -	**cal**	
Total ounces of water with meal -	**ounces**	
Total sodium of meal -	**mgs**	

Time of meal 4 - ________

Food eaten- ____

Drink - ________________________

Carbohydrates	**Protein**	**Fat**
Total crab grams -	Total protein grams -	Total fat grams -
Total fiber grams -		
Total sugar grams -		
Total complex grams -		
Total calories of meal -	**cal**	
Total ounces of water with meal -	**ounces**	
Total sodium of meal -	**mgs**	

Time of meal 5 - ________

Food eaten- ____

Drink - ________________________

Carbohydrates	**Protein**	**Fat**
Total crab grams -	Total protein grams -	Total fat grams -
Total fiber grams -		
Total sugar grams -		
Total complex grams -		
Total calories of meal -	**cal**	
Total ounces of water with meal -	**ounces**	
Total sodium of meal -	**mgs**	

Total ounces of water with meals - ounces
Total ounces of water during workout - ounces
Total ounces of water outside meals - ounces
Total ounces of water today - ounces
Total sodium today - mgs

Round 5 is in the bag; almost. Tomorrow is Day 7 and it's your day off, but there are a few things I want you to start doing on the evenings before your workout days. I want you to take about 5-10 minutes and look over your workout for the next day, and take a look at that same workout in the appendix in the back of the book. If you want, you can even start writing the weights you think you'll be using for each exercise into your workout log for the next day. If it ends up being a different weight when you actually do it, so what; just put a line through it and write the right weight down. Now go eat, sleep, or whatever else it is you do on this day; just make it something good.

Round 5 - *Day 7*

Great job on Round 5! As usual, you can record a heart rate if you want and journal your food if it helps you to stay on course, or you can simply do nothing. I like nothing sometimes, but it often ends up being something for my hyper self. Remember to take a look at your workout for tomorrow and if you want, go ahead and write down the weight amounts you think you'll be using for each exercise, or at least the first few sets. Whatever you do today, make sure it ends with a head full of positive thoughts, some good clean food, and a great night's sleep. I'll see you on Round 6!

Day 7 HR ______ Time taken _______

Food Journal

Time of meal 1 - _________

Food eaten- ____

Drink - ________________________

Carbohydrates	**Protein**	**Fat**
Total crab grams -	Total protein grams -	Total fat grams -
Total fiber grams -		
Total sugar grams -		
Total complex grams -		

Total calories of meal - cal
Total ounces of water with meal - ounces
Total sodium of meal - mgs

Time of meal 2 - _________

Food eaten- ____

Drink - ________________________

Carbohydrates	**Protein**	**Fat**
Total crab grams -	Total protein grams -	Total fat grams -
Total fiber grams -		
Total sugar grams -		
Total complex grams -		
Total calories of meal -	**cal**	
Total ounces of water with meal -	**ounces**	
Total sodium of meal -	**mgs**	

Time of meal 3 (Lunch) - _________

Food eaten- ____

Drink - ________________________

Carbohydrates	**Protein**	**Fat**
Total crab grams -	Total protein grams -	Total fat grams -
Total fiber grams -		
Total sugar grams -		
Total complex grams -		
Total calories of meal -	**cal**	
Total ounces of water with meal -	**ounces**	
Total sodium of meal -	**mgs**	

Time of meal 4 - _________

Food eaten- ____

Drink - ________________________

Carbohydrates	**Protein**	**Fat**
Total crab grams -	Total protein grams -	Total fat grams -
Total fiber grams -		
Total sugar grams -		
Total complex grams -		
Total calories of meal -	**cal**	
Total ounces of water with meal -	**ounces**	
Total sodium of meal -	**mgs**	

Time of meal 5 - _________

Food eaten- ____

Drink - ________________________

Carbohydrates	**Protein**	**Fat**
Total crab grams -	Total protein grams -	Total fat grams -
Total fiber grams -		
Total sugar grams -		
Total complex grams -		

Total calories of meal - cal
Total ounces of water with meal - ounces
Total sodium of meal - mgs

Total ounces of water with meals - ounces
Total ounces of water outside meals - ounces
Total ounces of water today - ounces
Total sodium today - mgs

Round 6 – Building Your Health Portfolio

Day 1

It's hard for me to believe, but here we are for Round 6. Here's the deal: Round 6 is the point where many things start to change like your strength and endurance, getting closer to reaching your goals, being more specific with visualization, and a very detailed food journal. Round 6 is more of a transition round to the second half of 12 Rounds because starting with Round 7, this entire program ramps up and you will be challenged in every way possible. But don't worry; I'm going to be there every step you take and from what I've seen in you, I might just have a problem keeping up. It's time for Round 6; finish this first half strong, and go make it yours!

"Many people invest in stocks, real estate, and precious metals, but they're missing the most important investment of all. Mobility is the Real Gold!" ***Bobby Whisnand***

It Happened Just Like This!

I was presenting to a bank in Dallas last year and the first words I said to them were, "As individuals, at what point in your life does your mobility become more important than your money?" They were definitely not expecting to hear that question. Sure, it's important to plan for your future by saving and investing your money, but what about the other thing you're going to need in your future, are you planning for it too? You can have all the money in the world, but if you aren't able to enjoy it because your body and joints are worn out and you heart isn't strong enough to support you very well, what quality of life will you really have?"

I'm going to ask you the same question: At what point in your life does your mobility become more important than your money? I hope you said "NOW" because that's not only the right answer, it's the only answer. Let's go get this Round 6!

That One Thing

Take one minute right now and think about how you want to be able to live the rest of your life, especially when you retire. I'm not talking about money or lifestyle; I'm talking about being as active as you want to be and being able to have energy, strength, endurance, and unlimited mobility.

Write down one "Bucket List" thing you want to do later in your life or once you retire.

____

Seeing I to Eye

If you have pain in your body like in your back, knees, hips, shoulders, or anywhere else, take 4-5 minutes today and visualize yourself pain free. It's challenging but you can do it. Regardless of whether or not you have pain, visualize being active and doing something vigorous like climbing, running, playing a sport, or anything requiring full mobility. Now, do the things today that will ensure you will be active for the rest of your life and be able to do the very things you pictured.

Your Workout – See your workout log for today's workout

And the Heart Says…

Tonight when you are lying in bed and before you go to sleep, take one more heart rate and write it down here.

Pre Sleep HR - ______ Time taken ________

Cleaning Your Plate

One of the biggest mistakes made when starting to eat better is cutting out too many calories. While it's true you're more than likely going to cut some calories, you want to make sure you're getting enough to support your lean muscles and to provide enough energy for your body. The amount of calories and the type of calories you need is based on many variables which makes it impossible for me to give you the exact amount you need without knowing your goals and current condition. But coming up next week, we are going to start counting total calories for carbohydrates, proteins, and fats for each meal. In addition, I'm going to give you a ratio of what these should be within your diet.

You Ate What???

For this week, I want you to continue evaluating two meals a day, mark them accordingly, and log your sodium intakes for all meals. I know this is a lot but this entire food journal will help you for the rest of your life.

Food Journal

Time of meal 1 - _________

Food eaten- ____

Drink - ________________________

Carbohydrates	**Protein**	**Fat**
Total crab grams -	Total protein grams -	Total fat grams -
Total fiber grams -		
Total sugar grams -		
Total complex grams -		

Total calories of meal - **cal**
Total ounces of water with meal - **ounces**
Total sodium of meal - **mgs**

Time of meal 2 - _________

Food eaten- ____

Drink - ________________________

Carbohydrates	**Protein**	**Fat**
Total crab grams -	Total protein grams -	Total fat grams -
Total fiber grams -		
Total sugar grams -		
Total complex grams -		

Total calories of meal - **cal**
Total ounces of water with meal - **ounces**
Total sodium of meal - **mgs**

Time of meal 3 (Lunch) - _________

Food eaten- ____

Drink - ________________________

Carbohydrates	**Protein**	**Fat**
Total crab grams -	Total protein grams -	Total fat grams -
Total fiber grams -		
Total sugar grams -		
Total complex grams -		

Total calories of meal - **cal**
Total ounces of water with meal - **ounces**
Total sodium of meal - **mgs**

Time of meal 4 - _________

Food eaten- ____

Drink - ________________________

Carbohydrates	**Protein**	**Fat**
Total crab grams -	Total protein grams -	Total fat grams -
Total fiber grams -		
Total sugar grams -		
Total complex grams -		

Total calories of meal - **cal**
Total ounces of water with meal - **ounces**
Total sodium of meal - **mgs**

Time of meal 5 - _________

Food eaten- ____

Drink - ________________________

Carbohydrates	**Protein**	**Fat**
Total crab grams -	Total protein grams -	Total fat grams -
Total fiber grams -		
Total sugar grams -		
Total complex grams -		

Total calories of meal - **cal**
Total ounces of water with meal - **ounces**
Total sodium of meal - **mgs**

Total ounces of water with meals - **ounces**
Total ounces of water during workout - **ounces**
Total ounces of water outside meals - **ounces**
Total ounces of water today - **ounces**
Total sodium today - **mgs**

Great job Champ! It's the end to a productive day for you, and now it's time for you to relax, watch your favorite show on T.V., and go dream BIG! I'm not going anywhere; well, maybe to the refrigerator.

Round 6 - Day 2

Hello Day 2! Today is your core and cardio day so fuel up, round up, and let's get going!

Which Way You Headed?

So far you have two long term goals about something other than your fitness. Today, let's write these two goals here again and while you're at it, add a third goal.

My first two long term goals about something other than my fitness are…

Goal 1 - ____

Goal 2 - ____

My third long term (7 week) goal about something other than my fitness is…

Goal 3 -____

Seeing I to Eye

Think about your first long term goal that's about something other than fitness and take 4-5 minutes today and visualize yourself reaching that goal. When you get that picture in your mind, be as specific as you can with your visualization so your mind can better understand exactly what it is you want.

Upper Management

Did you print that list of things to do and put it where you can see it every day? If you did, great! Take a look at it today and find another thing you need to do and make a plan to check it off. If you didn't, make it a point to print it out today and place it where you can see it. We are really going to move on this so catch up before you get too far behind. The more you check off, the less stress you'll have.

Your Workout – See your workout log for today's workout.

Cleaning Your Plate

Why do you need to eat 4-5 smaller meals a day vs. 2-3 larger meals? The two main goals with weight management are as follows: The first is to give your body the exact amount of the right kinds of calories that your body will burn off on any given day without having any leftover; this is the calories in vs. calories out approach. The other goal with weight management is to give your body the right amount and the right kinds of calories **at the right times**; this is where eating 4-5 smaller meals a day is the most efficient. If you eat too many calories at once, your body and its metabolism will slow down and more than likely store the excess nutrition you gave it as body fat. But if you eat smaller amounts throughout your day, your body can easily breakdown and consume the calories for energy without slowing everything down which raises your metabolism. Does this make sense to you? Please say yes.

You Ate What???

As you journal your food this week, take notice to how many meals you are eating a day. If it's just 2-3, start thinking about ways to spread these out into 4-5 meals a day. Remember, these aren't all big meals; two of your meals a day can be things like a protein drink, fruit, and some nuts.

Food Journal

Time of meal 1 - _________

Food eaten- ____

Drink - ________________________

Carbohydrates	**Protein**	**Fat**
Total crab grams -	Total protein grams -	Total fat grams -
Total fiber grams -		
Total sugar grams -		
Total complex grams -		

Total calories of meal - cal
Total ounces of water with meal - ounces
Total sodium of meal - mgs

Time of meal 2 - _________

Food eaten- ____

Drink - ________________________

Carbohydrates	**Protein**	**Fat**
Total crab grams -	Total protein grams -	Total fat grams -
Total fiber grams -		
Total sugar grams -		
Total complex grams -		

Total calories of meal - cal
Total ounces of water with meal - ounces
Total sodium of meal - mgs

Time of meal 3 (Lunch) - _________

Food eaten- ____

Drink - ________________________

Carbohydrates	**Protein**	**Fat**
Total crab grams -	Total protein grams -	Total fat grams -
Total fiber grams -		
Total sugar grams -		
Total complex grams -		

Total calories of meal - cal
Total ounces of water with meal - ounces
Total sodium of meal - mgs

Time of meal 4 - _________

Food eaten- ____

Drink - ________________________

Carbohydrates	**Protein**	**Fat**
Total crab grams -	Total protein grams -	Total fat grams -
Total fiber grams -		
Total sugar grams -		
Total complex grams -		
Total calories of meal -	**cal**	
Total ounces of water with meal -	**ounces**	
Total sodium of meal -	**mgs**	

Time of meal 5 - _________

Food eaten- ____

Drink - ________________________

Carbohydrates	**Protein**	**Fat**
Total crab grams -	Total protein grams -	Total fat grams -
Total fiber grams -		
Total sugar grams -		
Total complex grams -		
Total calories of meal -	**cal**	
Total ounces of water with meal -	**ounces**	
Total sodium of meal -	**mgs**	

Total ounces of water with meals - **ounces**
Total ounces of water during workout - **ounces**
Total ounces of water outside meals - **ounces**
Total ounces of water today - **ounces**
Total sodium today - **mgs**

And The Heart Says…
At some point in the middle of your day, take a heart rate and record it here.

Afternoon HR-________ Time taken - _______

You may not believe this, but if you are exercising just like I teach you with 12 Rounds, you're exercising better than 95% of the people I see every day. That's right! And if you're cleaning up your eating, reducing stress, and keeping positive things in that beautiful mind of yours, your life is changing right before your very eyes, and in a very good way. Sleep tight; I'll see you tomorrow.

Round 6 – Day 3

Oh yes! It's that day I love the most; LEG DAY. And even better than that; it's HEAVY LEG DAY! If you didn't take a look at the appendix in the back to get a gauge on how much weight you'll be using, go ahead and do it as soon as you can before your workout today; it will save you a lot of time. Okay, show off, let's get this day going.

That One Thing

Write down one way 12 Rounds is helping you invest in your future that has to do with improving and preserving your mobility so you'll have it for the rest of your life.

Seeing I to Eye

Think about your first long term goal that's about your fitness. Take 4-5 minutes today and visualize yourself reaching that goal. Make it real by adding sounds, colors, feelings, other people, and anything else to make it real. Remember to be as specific as you can.

Your Workout – See your workout log for today's workout.

***Shortened Workout** – This is one of the longest workouts you'll do simply because it's a unilateral heavy workout. If you have time constraints, do the workout in **bold** instead.

And the Heart Says…

At any point today after your workout and after you have been sitting for at least 3-4 minutes, take a resting heart rate and record it here.

Resting HR - ______ Time Taken - ________

Cleaning Your Plate

What makes processed foods so bad? There are two main reasons why food companies process foods: The first is to make it taste better and the second is to make it last longer. To do this, processed foods are manipulated or changed in the following ways:

- Adding sugar or high fructose corn syrup
- Adding artificial ingredients because it's cheaper for the manufacturer
- Adding trans fats and processed vegetable oils

Here are a few other characteristics of processed foods:

- Low in vitamins and minerals
- Low in fiber
- Processed foods digest quicker and require less energy to do so; cheap nutrition

Either way you look at it, processed foods are low in nutrients and full of things your body cannot use very well. This makes for a very cheap and unhealthy source of "food".

Do you know what one of the biggest sources of processed foods is? Baked Sweet Goods.

Read those labels!

You Ate What???

How are you doing with getting 4-5 smaller meals a day? Also, take a look at the foods you're eating and notice how many of them are sweets like candy, cakes, desserts, sodas, and other sweet foods. Now's the time to make your move away from these health destroying foods. I know they taste good, but they'll kill your body from the inside out.

Food Journal

Time of meal 1 - _________

Food eaten- ____

Drink - ________________________

Carbohydrates	**Protein**	**Fat**
Total crab grams -	Total protein grams -	Total fat grams -
Total fiber grams -		
Total sugar grams -		
Total complex grams -		

Total calories of meal - **cal**
Total ounces of water with meal - **ounces**
Total sodium of meal - **mgs**

Time of meal 2 - _________

Food eaten- ____

Drink - ________________________

Carbohydrates	**Protein**	**Fat**
Total crab grams -	Total protein grams -	Total fat grams -
Total fiber grams -		
Total sugar grams -		
Total complex grams -		

Total calories of meal - **cal**
Total ounces of water with meal - **ounces**
Total sodium of meal - **mgs**

Time of meal 3 (Lunch) - _________

Food eaten- ____

Drink - ________________________

Carbohydrates	**Protein**	**Fat**
Total crab grams -	Total protein grams -	Total fat grams -
Total fiber grams -		
Total sugar grams -		
Total complex grams -		

Total calories of meal - cal
Total ounces of water with meal - ounces
Total sodium of meal - mgs

Time of meal 4 - _________

Food eaten- ____

Drink - ________________________

Carbohydrates	**Protein**	**Fat**
Total crab grams -	Total protein grams -	Total fat grams -
Total fiber grams -		
Total sugar grams -		
Total complex grams -		

Total calories of meal - cal
Total ounces of water with meal - ounces
Total sodium of meal - mgs

Time of meal 5 - _________

Food eaten- ____

Drink - ________________________

Carbohydrates	**Protein**	**Fat**
Total crab grams -	Total protein grams -	Total fat grams -
Total fiber grams -		
Total sugar grams -		
Total complex grams -		

Total calories of meal - cal
Total ounces of water with meal - ounces
Total sodium of meal - mgs

Total ounces of water with meals - ounces
Total ounces of water during workout - ounces
Total ounces of water outside meals - ounces
Total ounces of water today - ounces
Total sodium today - mgs

Leg Day has come and gone but we still have two more workouts this week, and the best way to get ready for one is to recuperate from another. As I have said before, training legs takes a lot out of your body so make sure you are eating good unprocessed foods which help you recuperate faster. Better food, better body, better life. Oh yea, don't forget to add sleep in there too. Great job today!

Round 6 - Day 4

Today's the day where you get to give your body a break. You've been working out for three days straight and even though you may not feel it, your body needs a break. Your body and everything about it has a shelf life and I want yours to be the longest possible, so take it easy today, eat well, keep those thoughts positive and productive, and enjoy Day 4.

"Tax returns show how good or bad you did with your money each year; your joints and doctor bills tell you how good or bad you did taking care of yourself." ***Bobby Whisnand***

It Happened Just Like This!

One of my most memorable presentations happened at an accounting firm a few years ago. I got all of them involved in the following conversation: "Tell me if I'm wrong, but isn't it your main job as an accountant to take all of the financial information from your clients, crunch all the numbers, and then tell them where their money went, where their money needs to go, what tax they owe or will get in a return, and an overall assessment of their wealth?" I then said something that threw all of them for a loop. "The absolute best advice you could give your clients to help them manage their money for their future is the same advice that most, if not all of you are leaving out – advising your clients to invest in healthy exercise and healthy eating so that when they retire and get older, the chances of them spending their life's savings paying for someone else to take care of them becomes much less."

I can't tell you how many accountants came up to me after my presentation was over and told me I had definitely opened their eyes. I hope I've done the same for you my friend because investing in your health in the right ways now will get you a lot further than any amount of money ever will. The thing to remember is just like with investing your money, you have to make the right investments in your body today, so you'll still have a healthy body to use later in life.

Which Way You Headed?

So far you have two long term goals about your fitness. Today, let's write these two goals here again and while you're at it, add a third goal.

My first two long term goals about my fitness are:

Goal 1 - ____

Goal 2 - ____

My third long term (7 week) goal about my fitness is:

Goal 3 - ____

Seeing I to Eye

Think about your first long term goal about your fitness. Take 4-5 minutes today and visualize yourself reaching that goal. To really see yourself better than you currently are takes time and practice so don't get discouraged if it's taking some time for you to really "see" it. Believe me; your brain is listening so keep at it!

Upper Management

Did you print that list of things to do and put it where you can see it every day? If you did, great! Take a look at it today and find yet another thing you need to do and make a plan to check it off. If you didn't, take a minute right now and print it out so you can get going on it. It's pretty dang neat to see that list get shorter and shorter. But you have to be the one that starts it and finishes it. You've got this!

No Workout Today! Enjoy your day off

And the Heart Says...

Take at least one heart rate today whenever you want. Just make sure you write down when and under what circumstances you took it.

Today I took my heart rate when I was... ____

Day 4 HR - ______ Time taken - ________

Cleaning Your Plate

Let's face it; fast food is very tempting for several reasons: It's super convenient because it's on and around every corner, it's quick and easy, it's inexpensive, and it definitely tastes good. Your absolute best weapon and deterrent of eating fast food is to make and plan your meals ahead of time. Here's what I do and have been doing for a long time now with my food: On Sunday, I make enough food for three days and then on Wednesday, I make enough food for three more days. You can do the same things, and if you compare apples to apples, you'll more than likely save a ton of money as well. You can then take a small cooler to work with you and simply warm up your lunch and also have your other smaller meals in your cooler and ready to eat as well. I know what you're thinking; this takes time. You're right. It does take time, but this is one sure way you can nail down your eating and know for sure you're getting good clean food. Have I convinced you yet? That's okay; I've got six more weeks.

You Ate What???

As I mentioned earlier, it's impossible to tell you how many calories you should have a day without knowing everything about you, but you can add them up for yourself. If you're trying to lose weight, start reducing the carbohydrate and fat calories first and leave the protein calories alone. We will be getting into this next week so hang tight. The main thing is that you record any and all changes you're making to your eating so you'll know exactly where you are at any time.

Food Journal

Time of meal 1 - _________

Food eaten- ____

Drink - ________________________

Carbohydrates
Total crab grams -
Total fiber grams -
Total sugar grams -
Total complex grams -

Protein
Total protein grams -

Fat
Total fat grams -

Total calories of meal - cal
Total ounces of water with meal - ounces
Total sodium of meal - mgs

Time of meal 2 - _________

Food eaten- ____

Drink - ________________________

Carbohydrates	**Protein**	**Fat**
Total crab grams -	Total protein grams -	Total fat grams -
Total fiber grams -		
Total sugar grams -		
Total complex grams -		
Total calories of meal -	**cal**	
Total ounces of water with meal -	**ounces**	
Total sodium of meal -	**mgs**	

Time of meal 3 (Lunch) - _________

Food eaten- ____

Drink - ________________________

Carbohydrates	**Protein**	**Fat**
Total crab grams -	Total protein grams -	Total fat grams -
Total fiber grams -		
Total sugar grams -		
Total complex grams -		
Total calories of meal -	**cal**	
Total ounces of water with meal -	**ounces**	
Total sodium of meal -	**mgs**	

Time of meal 4 - _________

Food eaten- ____

Drink - ________________________

Carbohydrates	**Protein**	**Fat**
Total crab grams -	Total protein grams -	Total fat grams -
Total fiber grams -		
Total sugar grams -		
Total complex grams -		
Total calories of meal -	**cal**	
Total ounces of water with meal -	**ounces**	
Total sodium of meal -	**mgs**	

Time of meal 5 - _________

Food eaten- ____

Drink - ________________________

Carbohydrates	**Protein**	**Fat**
Total crab grams -	Total protein grams -	Total fat grams -
Total fiber grams -		
Total sugar grams -		
Total complex grams -		

Total calories of meal - **cal**
Total ounces of water with meal - **ounces**
Total sodium of meal - **mgs**

Total ounces of water with meals - **ounces**
Total ounces of water outside meals - **ounces**
Total ounces of water today - **ounces**
Total sodium today - **mgs**

Did you enjoy your day off from working out? I hope so because it's exactly what you need to keep yourself from overtraining. Now your body is rested and ready for a great back and bicep workout tomorrow. While I'm thinking about it; are you keeping track of how much water you're drinking a day? Make sure you are and take a look at it to see if you're getting enough. And make sure you get 10-12 ounces as soon as you get up in the mornings. See you tomorrow for back and biceps!

Round 6 - Day 5

How was your night? Did you get enough sleep? If you didn't, try taking a 15-20 minute nap today at some point, but don't get caught sleeping on the job; just be good at hiding. One thing I want you to pay particular attention to this morning is your water intake. Take a little extra notice to how much water you're drinking before noon today. I'll even put a place for you to record it. I know; I'm nice like that.

The total amount of water I drank today before noon was _______ounces.

That One Thing

Answer this one question for me: Are you treating your body now, how you want it to treat you later in life? Take a minute and think about your lifestyle, what you eat and drink, how you manage your stress, and how you exercise, and spend a little time today thinking how this affects your body in good or bad ways.

Seeing I to Eye

Here's a curve ball for you: Take a few minutes today and visualize how you want to look in 10 years. How's that for a picture? This is a fun one so have a good time with it but as always, keep it positive!

Your Workout – See your workout log for today's workout.

And the Heart Says…

Some time tonight after dinner and when you have been relaxing for about an hour, take and record a heart rate.

Evening resting HR ______ Time taken ______

Cleaning Your Plate

Starting with Round 7, we are going to add the last few steps to your food journal. The two things we're going to add is total calories for protein, carbs, and fats for each meal and the other thing we're going to add is to start balancing all of this out so you're eating the right amounts of each type of nutrition. By the way, carbs, proteins, and fats are often referred to as macronutrients in case you hear this label flying around.

To give you a head start, I want to give you a good macronutrient ratio for which to shoot with your diet. An ideal ratio of carbs/protein/fats is 40:30:30 which means your total daily caloric intake should be 40% carbs, 30% protein, and 30% fat. In my opinion, if you're goal is to drop some body fat, I would shoot for 30% carbs, 40% protein, and 30% fat. Don't worry about these today; we will discuss more later in Round 7.

You Ate What???

Keep journaling everything the same way for now' we'll add the things I mentioned above in Round 7.

Food Journal

Time of meal 1 - _________

Food eaten- ____

Drink - ________________________

Carbohydrates	**Protein**	**Fat**
Total carb grams -	Total protein grams -	Total fat grams -
Total fiber grams -		
Total sugar grams -		
Total complex grams -		
Total calories of meal -	**cal**	
Total ounces of water with meal -	**ounces**	
Total sodium of meal -	**mgs**	

Time of meal 2 - _________

Food eaten- ____

Drink - ________________________

Carbohydrates	**Protein**	**Fat**
Total carb grams -	Total protein grams -	Total fat grams -
Total fiber grams -		
Total sugar grams -		
Total complex grams -		
Total calories of meal -	**cal**	
Total ounces of water with meal -	**ounces**	
Total sodium of meal -	**mgs**	

Time of meal 3 (Lunch) - _________

Food eaten- ____

Drink - ________________________

Carbohydrates	**Protein**	**Fat**
Total carb grams -	Total protein grams -	Total fat grams -
Total fiber grams -		
Total sugar grams -		
Total complex grams -		

Total calories of meal - **cal**
Total ounces of water with meal - **ounces**
Total sodium of meal - **mgs**

Time of meal 4 - _________

Food eaten- ____

Drink - ________________________

Carbohydrates	**Protein**	**Fat**
Total carb grams -	Total protein grams -	Total fat grams -
Total fiber grams -		
Total sugar grams -		
Total complex grams -		

Total calories of meal - **cal**
Total ounces of water with meal - **ounces**
Total sodium of meal - **mgs**

Time of meal 5 - _________

Food eaten- ____

Drink - ________________________

Carbohydrates	**Protein**	**Fat**
Total carb grams -	Total protein grams -	Total fat grams -
Total fiber grams -		
Total sugar grams -		
Total complex grams -		

Total calories of meal - **cal**
Total ounces of water with meal - **ounces**
Total sodium of meal - **mgs**

Total ounces of water with meals - **ounces**
Total ounces of water during workout - **ounces**
Total ounces of water outside meals - **ounces**
Total ounces of water today - **ounces**
Total sodium today - **mgs**

Are you thinking what I'm thinking? I'm thinking about ice cream, brownies, and….just kidding! Well, maybe a little, but we're strong enough to stay away from those right? This has been another great day for you with another one coming up tomorrow. You know the drill; core and cardio are in store for tomorrow's workout so get your rest, keep that food clean, and let's get ready for a great weekend.

Round 6 - Day 6

Good news! We get to burn some of that body fat today. Are you ready for it? One key thing to burning body fat is to make sure you have the right nutrition in your body at the right times, especially before and after your workout. Make sure you are eating 1.5-2.5 hours before every workout so the food you ate has had time to turn into burning hot fuel. Let's go get it done!

Which Way You Headed?

So far you have two long term goals about your career. Today, let's write these two goals here again and while you're at it, add a third career goal.

My first two long term goals about my career are:

Goal 1 - ____

Goal 2 - ____

My third long term (7 week) goal about my career is:

Goal 3 - ____

Upper Management

We all have that old friend or family member with which we have lost touch. Maybe it's been several years or just a few months but either way, it's great when you reconnect and talk about old times isn't it? Over the next two days, reach out to one person with whom you have lost touch; it will make their day and yours a whole lot better.

Seeing I to Eye

Yesterday I asked you to visualize how you'll look in 10 years. Today, I want you to visualize how you want to look in 20 years. It's kind of funny and maybe even a little hard to do but give it a shot and see what you see. Remember, what you think is very powerful so make sure you see yourself healthy, active, and looking good! Just not as good as I'll look.

Your Workout – See your workout log for today's workout

And the Heart Says…

At some point this evening when you are relaxed, take another heart rate and record it here.

Post workout evening HR ______ Time taken __________

Cleaning Your Plate

What exactly are starchy carbs and what does it mean to your diet?

First of all, starchy carbs are found in foods like potatoes, legumes and beans, cereals, rice, grains, breads, and certain other vegetables. Believe it or not, there are many vegetables that are labeled as starchy carbs like corn, peas, parsnips, potatoes, pumpkin, squash, zucchini and yams. These are "starchy carbs" because they are more nutrient dense and contain more calories than a "non- starchy carb". You still need starchy carbs in your diet; you just have to consume a lower amount of these because they are higher in calories. What about non-starchy carbs; what exactly are they?

Non-starchy carbs are typically flowering parts of the plant like lettuce, asparagus, broccoli, cauliflower, cucumber, spinach, mushrooms, onions, peppers and tomatoes. Think about eating some of these and you will see why one is starchy and the other isn't; some are a lot denser than others like potatoes, right? You can keep track of these in your food journal too; just saying.

You Ate What???

We're getting closer to really making your food journal a piece of work. Yes, it contains a whole lot of information but the more of which we keep track, the better you'll know what to change to get your desired body composition. Keep looking at your total calories for each type of food; we're going to address this real quick.

Food Journal

Time of meal 1 - _________

Food eaten- ____

Drink - ________________________

Carbohydrates	**Protein**	**Fat**
Total carb grams -	Total protein grams -	Total fat grams -
Total fiber grams -		
Total sugar grams -		
Total complex grams -		
Total calories of meal -	**cal**	
Total ounces of water with meal -	**ounces**	
Total sodium of meal -	**mgs**	

Time of meal 2 - _________

Food eaten- ____

Drink - ________________________

Carbohydrates	**Protein**	**Fat**
Total carb grams -	Total protein grams -	Total fat grams -
Total fiber grams -		
Total sugar grams -		
Total complex grams -		
Total calories of meal -	**cal**	
Total ounces of water with meal -	**ounces**	
Total sodium of meal -	**mgs**	

Time of meal 3 (Lunch) - ________

Food eaten- ____

Drink - ________________________

Carbohydrates
Total carb grams -
Total fiber grams -
Total sugar grams -
Total complex grams -

Protein
Total protein grams -

Fat
Total fat grams -

Total calories of meal - **cal**
Total ounces of water with meal - **ounces**
Total sodium of meal - **mgs**

Time of meal 4 - ________

Food eaten- ____

Drink - ________________________

Carbohydrates
Total carb grams -
Total fiber grams -
Total sugar grams -
Total complex grams -

Protein
Total protein grams -

Fat
Total fat grams -

Total calories of meal - **cal**
Total ounces of water with meal - **ounces**
Total sodium of meal - **mgs**

Time of meal 5 - ________

Food eaten- ____

Drink - ________________________

Carbohydrates
Total carb grams -
Total fiber grams -
Total sugar grams -
Total complex grams -

Protein
Total protein grams -

Fat
Total fat grams -

Total calories of meal - **cal**
Total ounces of water with meal - **ounces**
Total sodium of meal - **mgs**

Total ounces of water with meals - **ounces**
Total ounces of water during workout - **ounces**
Total ounces of water outside meals - **ounces**
Total ounces of water today - **ounces**
Total sodium today - **mgs**

How are those abs feeling? I know you didn't do much in the way of cardio activity today but if you look at your workout results like average heart rates and calories burned, you'll see that just because you're not doing "cardio like" activity such as the treadmill, running, and cycling, you're still getting aerobic conditioning. The same holds true for your weekly weight training, especially those "light" days. I'll talk more about this over the next six weeks, but for now, let's close out this day with good food, good thoughts, and a night full of good dream filled sleep. See you tomorrow!

Round 6 - Day 7

Hey Champ, how are you feeling today? Me? I'm feeling great because I know what's in store for you over the next six weeks. That's right; you're exactly half way through 12 Rounds and boy let me tell you; things are going to take off big time for you over the next half of this program and you're going to see changes like you've never seen before; both physically and mentally. Making progress with your body is awesome, but when you add improving your mind, your confidence, and your outlook on life, anything is possible for you. Let's finish this Day 7 and get ready for the best of 12 Rounds starting tomorrow!

I took this heart rate when I was...____

Day 7 HR ______ Time taken _______

Food Journal

Time of meal 1 - _________

Food eaten- ____

Drink - ________________________

Carbohydrates	**Protein**	**Fat**
Total carb grams -	Total protein grams -	Total fat grams -
Total fiber grams -		
Total sugar grams -		
Total complex grams -		
Total calories of meal -	**cal**	
Total ounces of water with meal -	**ounces**	
Total sodium of meal -	**mgs**	

Time of meal 2 - _________

Food eaten- ____

Drink - ________________________

Carbohydrates	**Protein**	**Fat**
Total carb grams -	Total protein grams -	Total fat grams -
Total fiber grams -		
Total sugar grams -		
Total complex grams -		
Total calories of meal -	**cal**	
Total ounces of water with meal -	**ounces**	
Total sodium of meal -	**mgs**	

Time of meal 3 (Lunch) - _________

Food eaten- ____

Drink - ________________________

Carbohydrates	**Protein**	**Fat**
Total carb grams -	Total protein grams -	Total fat grams -
Total fiber grams -		
Total sugar grams -		
Total complex grams -		

Total calories of meal - **cal**
Total ounces of water with meal - **ounces**
Total sodium of meal - **mgs**

Time of meal 4 - _________

Food eaten- ____

Drink - ________________________

Carbohydrates	**Protein**	**Fat**
Total carb grams -	Total protein grams -	Total fat grams -
Total fiber grams -		
Total sugar grams -		
Total complex grams -		

Total calories of meal - **cal**
Total ounces of water with meal - **ounces**
Total sodium of meal - **mgs**

Time of meal 5 - _________

Food eaten- ____

Drink - ________________________

Carbohydrates	**Protein**	**Fat**
Total carb grams -	Total protein grams -	Total fat grams -
Total fiber grams -		
Total sugar grams -		
Total complex grams -		

Total calories of meal - **cal**
Total ounces of water with meal - **ounces**
Total sodium of meal - **mgs**

Total ounces of water with meals - **ounces**
Total ounces of water outside meals - **ounces**
Total ounces of water today - **ounces**
Total sodium today - **mgs**

The Second Half

Here you are at the exact half way mark of 12 Rounds. Can you believe it? As much as I can't wait to get you started on the second half, I want to list a few things for you to be aware of over the next six rounds. As I stated at the beginning of Round 6, the next six rounds are going to challenge you physically, mentally, and emotionally, but in very good and productive ways. We're going to start getting more specific with your goals, get more detailed with your visualization, become an expert at managing your stress, add more detail to your food journals, and last but not least, we're going to take your workouts to the next level.

I've used 12 Rounds for myself and all of my clients for the last several years and the number one thing that stands out to me with this program is that 12 Rounds works amazingly for every single person who uses it; as long as they use it exactly how it was designed. And the best thing is…they love doing it, and I hope you feel the same way. Before we move on to the second half, I'm going to give you a quick list of things I want you to do so you can make the next six rounds even better than the first ones. Are you ready?

- ➔ No matter where you go on any given day, always take 12 Rounds with you. As you know by now, 12 Rounds continuously builds from one day to the next so keep it close.
- ➔ Stick to 12 Rounds just like it says and if something happens and you miss a day; get right back on track the next day and don't look back.
- ➔ On your workout days, use these workouts exactly like they are designed in terms of sets, reps, rest time between sets, unilateral, reverse, and any other variables within the workouts. Don't do extra exercises or added cardio activity. If you do these workouts the way they are written, you definitely do not need to do anything else in exercise. I really am watching you.
- ➔ Do your absolute best to fill out your food journal every day as specifically as you can. The best part of these journals is you can use them for the rest of your life. Even if you made bad eating choices, write these down; it's all part of making progress. Even if it's really bad, I won't tell anyone.
- ➔ Stay on top of your goals and if you reach them early, write more goals to replace them.
- ➔ Make sure you are doing your *Pregame* before all workouts as well as *Finishing Strong* after your workouts. These make the biggest differences in any fitness program.
- ➔ Keep taking and recording those daily heart rates as well as your heart rates during your workouts. This is the single most telling indicator of just how healthy you really are.
- ➔ Be sure to communicate with that person or persons with whom you chose to share your goals and progresses with 12 Rounds. This is your support and as you know, there will be times when you need them. Keep them close.
- ➔ As hard as it may be on some days, keep visualizing positive things for yourself. Your mind will lead the way regardless of what you think so keep it positive.

That's it; these are the things I want you to keep in the front of your mind for the next six rounds so you can really hammer this thing home. Just in case you want to do your body measurements again or do them for the first time with 12 Rounds, I have a place below for you to record them. Again, you absolutely don't have to do it, but it's here if you want to.

Body Measurements

- **Date of measurements** - ___________________
- **Body weight** - _________ lbs
- **Body fat%** - ___________%
- **Shoulders** (measure across mid shoulder line) - _______
- **Chest** (measure across nipple line) - ________
- **Upper arm** (measure across mid bicep) - _______
- **Forearm** (measure across mid forearm between wrist and elbow) - _______
- **Waist** (measure right across belly button) - ________
- **Hips** (measure across mid buttocks) - ________
- **Upper thigh** (measure across mid upper thigh) - ________
- **Lower thigh** (measure across just above knee) - _______
- **Calf (**measure across mid calf) - _______

Round 7 – Wait Management

Day 1

Now we're really going to roll! Are you ready for the best six weeks in fitness and self improvement you've ever had? This is it! This is where your biggest gains in exercise, eating well, managing your stress, and overall feeling great about yourself are going to take place. I'm glad I get to be a part of it with you and see you take off like never before. One more thing: Be sure to pay close attention to your workout variables today and on all of your workout days because even though some of these workouts will seem familiar, they all have big differences. Let's do this!

"Some people spend so much of their lives waiting on things to happen that they let the really good things pass them by; like living." ***Bobby Whisnand***

It Happened Just Like This!

There's that old saying, "waiting is the hardest part", and boy is it right on! I learned a very hard lesson about seven years ago in business, and it was a tough one. I had just finished designing my *It's All Heart* fitness program and was ready for it to be filmed. The first two days of filming went so well, I just knew within the next 6 months, I would be in the market with my brand new fitness program. I told everyone it would be ready in six months, but little did I know; six months was about to turn into six years.

As it turned out, the way it was shot was very poor quality and we had no choice but to shoot the whole thing again. But again, bad quality was the result and all we really had was a week's worth of useless video. To make a long story short, I went through four different media companies to finally get it right. On top of that debacle, I went through five different web designers and three different business partners to finally get it right and in the market six years later.

One positive thing that happened to me during those very frustrating and disappointing years was that I got very good at managing my "wait." Even though it didn't happen the way I wanted it to or as fast as I wanted it to, it did finally happen, and I'm so glad I never gave up. Improving your health, career, personal life, finances, and other things will be challenging and just because things may not happen as fast as you'd like them to, isn't a reason to quit. Become good at managing your wait; it will pay off big time!

That One Thing

We all have things that test our patience, make us say bad words, pull our hair out, and bite our own teeth. The thing is those things will always be around in one form or another, so the best thing to do is to learn how to cope with it. Think about one of those things now without gritting your teeth and write it down here. Make it a good one!

One thing that absolutely drives me bat crazy that really tests my patience is…

____

Seeing I to Eye

I want you to think about a recent event in your life when you lost your patience and reacted not so well. Take 3-4 minutes today somewhere quiet and play that scene back in your mind except this time, visualize yourself having patience and not getting worked up. This might be a little sensitive for you but you can do it. Stay tough now.

And the Heart Says…

Let's see what your heart is doing outside of your exercise. Tonight when you're about to go to sleep, take a heart rate and record it here.

Pre Sleep HR - ______ Time taken ________

Cleaning Your Plate

Do you take a multi vitamin and mineral supplement?

I have people ask me this question a lot and I always give them the same answer: Absolutely I do. And so should you, unless your doctor has told you not to. When it comes to vitamin and mineral supplementation, it becomes even more important when you exercise on a regular basis because you use a lot more of these when your body is functioning at a higher level. In most cases, I always suggest a reputable vitamin and mineral supplement on a daily schedule, and depending on a person's activity level and exercise intensity, I also suggest higher doses of certain vitamins and minerals outside of a one-a-day type. With so many of us having different needs and health issues, I recommend you refer to your doctor or a registered dietician about this.

Here's a great source for you to use to determine if you should or should not take a vitamin and mineral supplement:

http://www.webmd.com/vitamins-and-supplements/lifestyle-guide-11/vitamins-minerals-how-much-should-you-take

You Ate What???

We're going to add a few things in a few days but for now, just keep doing what you're doing, as long as you're journaling everything that is.

Food Journal

Time of meal 1 - _________

Food eaten- ____

Drink - ________________________

Carbohydrates	**Protein**	**Fat**
Total carb grams -	Total protein grams -	Total fat grams -
Total fiber grams -		
Total sugar grams -		
Total complex grams -		
Total calories of meal -	**cal**	
Total ounces of water with meal -	**ounces**	
Total sodium of meal -	**mgs**	

Time of meal 2 - _________

Food eaten- ____

Drink - ________________________

Carbohydrates	**Protein**	**Fat**
Total carb grams -	Total protein grams -	Total fat grams -
Total fiber grams -		
Total sugar grams -		
Total complex grams -		
Total calories of meal -	**cal**	
Total ounces of water with meal -	**ounces**	
Total sodium of meal -	**mgs**	

Time of meal 3 (Lunch) - _________

Food eaten- ____

Drink - ________________________

Carbohydrates	**Protein**	**Fat**
Total carb grams -	Total protein grams -	Total fat grams -
Total fiber grams -		
Total sugar grams -		
Total complex grams -		
Total calories of meal -	**cal**	
Total ounces of water with meal -	**ounces**	
Total sodium of meal -	**mgs**	

Time of meal 4 - _________

Food eaten- ____

Drink - ________________________

Carbohydrates	**Protein**	**Fat**
Total carb grams -	Total protein grams -	Total fat grams -
Total fiber grams -		
Total sugar grams -		
Total complex grams -		
Total calories of meal -	**cal**	
Total ounces of water with meal -	**ounces**	
Total sodium of meal -	**mgs**	

Time of meal 5 - _________

Food eaten- ____

Drink - ________________________

Carbohydrates	**Protein**	**Fat**
Total carb grams -	Total protein grams -	Total fat grams -
Total fiber grams -		
Total sugar grams -		
Total complex grams -		

Total calories of meal - **cal**
Total ounces of water with meal - **ounces**
Total sodium of meal - **mgs**

Total ounces of water with meals - **ounces**
Total ounces of water during workout - **ounces**
Total ounces of water outside meals - **ounces**
Total ounces of water today - **ounces**
Total sodium today - **mgs**

That's what I'm talking about! A great start to the second half of 12 Rounds. Keep this momentum going because we're going to do some great things over the next six rounds. Tonight when you go to bed and right before you go to sleep, take a minute to clear your mind of all negative and stressful things, replace them with good thoughts, and wake up ready to take on the world. I'll be right there with you!

Round 7 - Day 2

This is your day! Regardless of anything else from this point forward; today is yours. Although many things are out of your control, there are plenty of things that are in your control like being on time and not having to rush, not letting little things bother you, keeping those stressful and irritating situations at a minimum, and smiling so the whole world can see it. Now go make it yours!

Which Way You Headed?

Lets' start this Round 7 goal setting with a little assessment of the goals to which you've already committed. Write your three goals about something other than fitness. For each goal, give an honest assessment of how much you have achieved to this point by giving a percentage. If you have reached any of these goals, go ahead and write another one to replace the ones you've reached.

My three long term goals about something other than fitness including my assessment to this point:

Goal 1 - ____

I feel I have reached ______% of this goal

Goal 2 - ____

I feel I have reached ______% of this goal

Goal 3 - ____

I feel I have reached ______% of this goal

Seeing I to Eye

Think of a hectic experience you've had recently. Once you got it in your head, visualize a better, more peaceful ending to the same experience. This one will take some concentration and good effort on your part so make sure you are in a quiet place with no distractions. Leave that phone behind!

Upper Management

Laughter is one of the best stress reducers in the world. Today, find a source of humor you can use during the week whether at work, home, or anywhere else. It might be a book of jokes, a funny book, or a funny article you can find on the internet. Either way, get a hold of it because we are going to use it over the next six weeks. That's your homework.

Your Workout – See your workout log for today's workout

Cleaning Your Plate

What are BCAAs and do you need to take them?

First of all, BCAAs stands for Branched-Chain Amino Acids and they are very popular in the world of exercise and especially body building. You can see people working out drinking their BCAAs in their water bottles or even in milk jugs throughout the course of their workouts. So, what's up with this? For the reason that this subject can get very detailed and comprehensive, I'm going to give you a basic breakdown of what BCAAs do and whether or not you should take them.

Branch Chain Amino Acids are the "Building Blocks" of the body. They make up 35% of your muscle mass and must be present for molecular growth and development to take place. Eight are essential (cannot be manufactured by the body) the rest are non-essential (can be manufactured by the body with proper nutrition). Besides building cells and repairing tissue, they form antibodies, and are part of the enzyme & hormonal system. They build RNA and DNA, and they carry oxygen throughout the body.

Now, should you take them or not?

The biggest proponent to taking BCAAs is to help you grow and keep lean muscle while you are trying to lose body fat. Getting your body to burn body fat is tricky, but once your body does start to burn body fat, there's a good chance you'll lose some muscle mass as well. This is where BCAAs help out by synthesizing protein fast enough to keep up with your body's need for energy while restricting calories. I think taking BCAAs is a good idea for most people who exercise. I like to think of it as insurance that my body isn't going to burn lean muscle mass as energy. I take them every day whether I'm working out or not, and from what I can tell, they definitely have a positive effect. If you do want to take them, drink them slowly across the duration of each workout you do, and don't forget to drink enough water as well.

You Ate What???

Keep taking a close look at the types and amounts of the food you're eating, place check marks by the good choices, and start making changes to those bad choices. I know this can seem to be tedious but these food journals are the making of something you will be able to use for the rest of your life. Keep at it; you will soon reap the rewards.

Food Journal

Time of meal 1 - _________

Food eaten- ____

Drink - ________________________

Carbohydrates	**Protein**	**Fat**
Total carb grams -	Total protein grams -	Total fat grams -
Total fiber grams -		
Total sugar grams -		
Total complex grams -		
Total calories of meal -	**cal**	
Total ounces of water with meal -	**ounces**	
Total sodium of meal -	**mgs**	

Time of meal 2 - _________

Food eaten- ____

Drink - ________________________

Carbohydrates	**Protein**	**Fat**
Total carb grams -	Total protein grams -	Total fat grams -
Total fiber grams -		
Total sugar grams -		
Total complex grams -		
Total calories of meal -	**cal**	
Total ounces of water with meal -	**ounces**	
Total sodium of meal -	**mgs**	

Time of meal 3 (Lunch) - _________

Food eaten- ____

Drink - ________________________

Carbohydrates	**Protein**	**Fat**
Total carb grams -	Total protein grams -	Total fat grams -
Total fiber grams -		
Total sugar grams -		
Total complex grams -		
Total calories of meal -	**cal**	
Total ounces of water with meal -	**ounces**	
Total sodium of meal -	**mgs**	

Time of meal 4 - _________

Food eaten- ____

Drink - ________________________

Carbohydrates
Total carb grams -
Total fiber grams -
Total sugar grams -
Total complex grams -

Protein
Total protein grams -

Fat
Total fat grams -

Total calories of meal - **cal**
Total ounces of water with meal - **ounces**
Total sodium of meal - **mgs**

Time of meal 5 - _________

Food eaten- ____

Drink - ________________________

Carbohydrates
Total carb grams -
Total fiber grams -
Total sugar grams -
Total complex grams -

Protein
Total protein grams -

Fat
Total fat grams -

Total calories of meal - **cal**
Total ounces of water with meal - **ounces**
Total sodium of meal - **mgs**

Total ounces of water with meals - **ounces**
Total ounces of water during workout - **ounces**
Total ounces of water outside meals - **ounces**
Total ounces of water today - **ounces**
Total sodium today - **mgs**

And The Heart Says…

At some point in the middle of your day, take a heart rate and record it here.

Afternoon HR-________ Time taken - _______

I hope this day was good my friend and that you gave it your best shot. Like I said at the beginning of this day, you can't control everything that's going to happen across the course of your day or your life, but you can control how you respond to it. Life has its challenges, tough times, and times where you may wonder if it's ever going to get better. This is where you have to fight to have a better life and do the things today that will help you face those tough times when they show up. Before you go to sleep tonight, put a smile on that face of yours because you are learning to live life on your terms, and that's an awesome way to live. Sleep tight and I'll see you tomorrow.

Round 7 – Day 3

Good morning! Are you ready for a kick butt leg day workout? I like leg day workouts the best because personally, they're the ones that typically are the most challenging, especially those light reverse workouts. Another reason I like leg day so much is that they make your entire body stronger, as long as you do them right. I know I've reminded you of this several times, but it can't be said enough: Make sure you are going slowly (4-5 seconds on every rep) and always using controlled movements during these workouts. Okay, enough of that; let's go do this!

That One Thing

On Day 1of this round, you wrote down one thing that tests your patience the most. Write it again here and this time, write down one thing you can do the next time this happens to help you be more patient.

One thing that really tests my patience is…

____

One thing I can do to handle this with patience the next time is…

____

Seeing I to Eye

Think of one thing that really relaxes you. It could be a massage, lying on the beach, walking a trail in the mountains, sitting in a park, or anything that really puts you at ease. Take 5 minutes today, get in that secluded place, and visualize you being there. I know where I'm going: Fishing!

Your Workout – See your workout log for today's workout.

And the Heart Says…

While you're at work today and sitting at your desk, take a heart rate and write it down here. Make sure you've been sitting for at least 5 minutes before you take it.

Resting HR - ______ Time Taken - ________

Cleaning Your Plate

Is it okay to drink meal replacement shakes instead of eating a solid meal?

One quick way to get good nutrition in your body is to drink shakes or meal replacement drinks. I think this is a great way to make sure you're getting enough good clean nutrition in your body but there are two ways this can be bad for you, so you have to be careful. First of all, your body's digestive process is designed around solid food. When you eat and are chewing food, this triggers other digestive functions in your stomach and it's all timed perfectly; most of the time that is. Once food is in your stomach, other digestive and absorption functions are taking place in your intestines and it's all based on timing. When you drink your nutrition, this timing can be thrown off and your absorption may not be as good as it is by eating solid food. Does that make sense?

The other way drinking your nutrition can be bad is when the contents or nutrition of the drink itself are of low quality. Make sure to read those labels including the ingredients so you'll not only know what kind of nutrition is in them, you'll also know the source of this nutrition.

I tell all of my clients to eat solid food for at least three of their 4-5 meals a day and only use meal replacement shakes once a day.

You Ate What???

Guess what? Yep; I'm going to add a few more things starting tomorrow so go ahead and take one more day and evaluate all of your meals, making marks where needed. You're becoming a food journaling pro aren't you? I know; exactly what you've always wanted to be.

Food Journal

Time of meal 1 - _________

Food eaten- ____

Drink - ________________________

Carbohydrates	**Protein**	**Fat**
Total carb grams -	Total protein grams -	Total fat grams -
Total fiber grams -		
Total sugar grams -		
Total complex grams -		
Total calories of meal -	**cal**	
Total ounces of water with meal -	**ounces**	
Total sodium of meal -	**mgs**	

Time of meal 2 - _________

Food eaten- ____

Drink - ________________________

Carbohydrates	**Protein**	**Fat**
Total carb grams -	Total protein grams -	Total fat grams -
Total fiber grams -		
Total sugar grams -		
Total complex grams -		
Total calories of meal -	**cal**	
Total ounces of water with meal -	**ounces**	
Total sodium of meal -	**mgs**	

Time of meal 3 (Lunch) - _________

Food eaten- ____

Drink - ________________________

Carbohydrates	**Protein**	**Fat**
Total carb grams -	Total protein grams -	Total fat grams -
Total fiber grams -		
Total sugar grams -		
Total complex grams -		

Total calories of meal - **cal**
Total ounces of water with meal - **ounces**
Total sodium of meal - **mgs**

Time of meal 4 - _________

Food eaten- ____

Drink - ________________________

Carbohydrates	**Protein**	**Fat**
Total carb grams -	Total protein grams -	Total fat grams -
Total fiber grams -		
Total sugar grams -		
Total complex grams -		

Total calories of meal - **cal**
Total ounces of water with meal - **ounces**
Total sodium of meal - **mgs**

Time of meal 5 - _________

Food eaten- ____

Drink - ________________________

Carbohydrates	**Protein**	**Fat**
Total carb grams -	Total protein grams -	Total fat grams -
Total fiber grams -		
Total sugar grams -		
Total complex grams -		

Total calories of meal - **cal**
Total ounces of water with meal - **ounces**
Total sodium of meal - **mgs**

Total ounces of water with meals - **ounces**
Total ounces of water during workout - **ounces**
Total ounces of water outside meals - **ounces**
Total ounces of water today - **ounces**
Total sodium today - **mgs**

That was a great day for you, and there's many more to come. One thing I want you to start doing on the evenings before your workout days is to spend a little time looking at Appendix A and writing down the weights you think you'll be using for your next workout. This is something I do every night or first thing the next morning before my workout. It will definitely save you a lot of time, especially on those lightening fast light days. Eat well, think great, and sleep like a bear. I'll see you tomorrow!

Round 7 - Day 4

Hey Champ! How did you sleep? Today is your day off from working out so no sneaking one in either; I'm counting on you. I've also got a great story for you to start your day; check it out.

"Is there a place on earth where the sun shines 24 hours a day? Yes, the sun is always shining; it's just a matter of if you can see it or not from where you currently are." **Bobby Whisnand**

It Happened Just Like This!

I have a friend who is probably the most impatient person I've ever known. I'll never forget the lake house he bought as a "project" to fix up and sell. When we opened the front door, it was so full of junk you could barely walk through the place. I urged him not to buy it because I knew he would end up being frustrated because it was going to take a while to empty that thing out. He ended up buying it anyway and after a month or so, I called him to see how it was going. He said, "Don't ask, it's a nightmare and I'm not even half way through. This has been nothing but a headache." I ended up getting several of my friends together to help him finish and we cleared that entire house out in two full days.

I think it's great to take on a big project but one thing you have to do is manage your expectations and don't give up when it takes longer than you had expected. It's all about "managing your wait" so you can enjoy the project instead of making yourself miserable. Go ahead and tackle something big; just be realistic, set your cruise control, and enjoy the ride.

Which Way You Headed?

Write your three goals about your fitness. For each goal, give an honest assessment of how much you have achieved to this point by giving a percentage. If you have reached any of these goals, go ahead and write another one to replace the ones you've reached.

My three long term goals about my fitness including my assessment to this point:

Goal 1 - ____

I feel I have reached ______% of this goal

Goal 2 - ____

I feel I have reached ______% of this goal

Goal 3 - ____

I feel I have reached ______% of this goal

Seeing I to Eye

Yesterday, you visualized something relaxing. Today, think of something else relaxing and go there for 4-5 minutes, but this time, make sure you add one of your favorite songs. Drinks with umbrellas are definitely advised.

Upper Management

On Day 2, you were to find a source of humor which you can use 3-4 days a week. Did you get that source? If you did, go ahead and take a few minutes to use it, and if you didn't, make it a point to get that source over the next two days. You don't want me telling jokes; it will either make you mad, or you'll just shake your head because it doesn't make any sense.

No Workout Today! Enjoy your day off

And the Heart Says…

Take at least one heart rate today whenever you want. Just make sure you write down when and under what circumstances you took it.

Today I took my heart rate when I was… ____

Day 4 HR - ______ Time taken - ________

Cleaning Your Plate

Take a close look at the ingredients on a few of the food items you have at home. Pay close attention to how long of a list it is. Typically, whole unprocessed foods have just a few ingredients where as processed foods have a list a mile long. Another thing you can do is to look up what some of those ingredients are because more than likely, there are preservatives and other chemicals to make it last longer.

You Ate What???

I want you to add just a few things to your food journal starting today. You're already recording total calories but now I want you to start breaking them down by recording total calories for carbs, proteins, and fats. The reason I want you to do this is because next week, we're going to put all of this together and start looking at the caloric ratios between your carbs, proteins, and fats. This is where you really start to nail things down.

Food Journal

Time of meal 1 - _________

Food eaten- ____

Drink - ________________________

Carbohydrates	**Protein**	**Fat**
Total carb grams -	Total protein grams -	Total fat grams -
Total fiber grams -	Total protein calories -	Total fat calories -
Total sugar grams -		
Total complex grams -		
Total carb calories -		

Total calories of meal - cal
Total ounces of water with meal - ounces
Total sodium of meal - mgs

Time of meal 2 - _________

Food eaten- ____

Drink - ________________________

Carbohydrates
Total carb grams -
Total fiber grams -
Total sugar grams -
Total complex grams -
Total carb calories -

Protein
Total protein grams -
Total protein calories -

Fat
Total fat grams -
Total fat calories -

Total calories of meal - **cal**
Total ounces of water with meal - **ounces**
Total sodium of meal - **mgs**

Time of meal 3 (Lunch) - _________

Food eaten- ____

Drink - ________________________

Carbohydrates
Total carb grams -
Total fiber grams -
Total sugar grams -
Total complex grams -
Total carb calories -

Protein
Total protein grams -
Total protein calories -

Fat
Total fat grams -
Total fat calories -

Total calories of meal - **cal**
Total ounces of water with meal - **ounces**
Total sodium of meal - **mgs**

Time of meal 4 - _________

Food eaten- ____

Drink - ________________________

Carbohydrates
Total carb grams -
Total fiber grams -
Total sugar grams -
Total complex grams -
Total carb calories -

Protein
Total protein grams -
Total protein calories -

Fat
Total fat grams -
Total fat calories -

Total calories of meal - **cal**
Total ounces of water with meal - **ounces**
Total sodium of meal - **mgs**

Time of meal 5 - ________

Food eaten- ____

Drink - ______________________

Carbohydrates	**Protein**	**Fat**
Total carb grams -	Total protein grams -	Total fat grams -
Total fiber grams -	Total protein calories -	Total fat calories -
Total sugar grams -		
Total complex grams -		
Total carb calories -		

Total calories of meal - **cal**
Total ounces of water with meal - **ounces**
Total sodium of meal - **mgs**

Total ounces of water with meals - **ounces**
Total ounces of water during workout - **ounces**
Total ounces of water outside meals - **ounces**
Total ounces of water today - **ounces**
Total sodium today - **mgs**

Now that's a food journal! Once you know the specifics of everything you eat and drink, you can make the right changes in your eating to get your desired results. It's chemistry at its best and you my friend are going to be a master chemist by the time I'm done with you. Oh yeah; make sure to look over your workout for tomorrow and Appendix A in the back so you can write down the weights you think you'll be using for each exercise. Enjoy the rest of your day and as always, keep positive things in that head of yours, and I'll see you tomorrow for back and biceps day.

Round 7 - Day 5

Oh yes; it's day 5 which means…It's Friday! If you didn't get a chance to write down your weights for today's workout, take some time today and do so; it will be well worth your time. How are you doing with your water intake these days? Make sure you're recording this in your food journal and don't forget that 10-12 ounces of water as soon as you get up. Back and Biceps here we come!

That One Thing

Think back to a time when you were impatient with your exercise and your health. Maybe it was losing weight, trying to get more energy, lower your blood pressure, or anything you were trying to accomplish by exercising and eating better and it became frustrating for you. Now write down one thing you have learned with 12 Rounds that has helped you manage your expectations with getting healthier.

One thing I have learned with 12 Rounds that has helped me manage my expectations with getting healthier is…

____

Seeing I to Eye

Let's get back to basics. Today, take 5 minutes to visualize yourself looking and feeling exactly like you want. This can be challenging but you are getting great at seeing exactly what you want to be, so go make it happen.

Your Workout – See your workout log for today's workout

And the Heart Says…

Sometime tonight after dinner and when you have been relaxing for about an hour, take and record a heart rate.

Evening resting HR ______ Time taken ______

Cleaning Your Plate

The Sweet Tooth! Oh yes; I've got a whole mouth full of those and if I didn't have a great way to fill the need, I would definitely be in trouble. If you have a sweet tooth, try drinking a protein drink to help curve your sweet cravings. There is a huge market for protein drinks, and if you'll ask, most health food and supplement stores have samples you can try to see which ones you like. The only thing you have to watch out for is the amount of "sugar" in some of these drinks. Make sure it has less than 3 grams of sugar and less than 8 grams of total carbs per serving. You know what you're doing at this point.

You Ate What???

Keep up the good work on your food journaling. Remember; we added total calories for carbs, proteins, and fats so keep up with those too. Also, keep a close eye on that sodium intake and do your best to stay at or below 1500mgs a day.

Food Journal

Time of meal 1 - _________

Food eaten- ____

Drink - ________________________

Carbohydrates	**Protein**	**Fat**
Total carb grams -	Total protein grams -	Total fat grams -
Total fiber grams -	Total protein calories -	Total fat calories -
Total sugar grams -		
Total complex grams -		
Total carb calories -		

Total calories of meal - cal
Total ounces of water with meal - ounces
Total sodium of meal - mgs

Time of meal 2 - _________

Food eaten- ____

Drink - ________________________

Carbohydrates	**Protein**	**Fat**
Total carb grams -	Total protein grams -	Total fat grams -
Total fiber grams -	Total protein calories -	Total fat calories -
Total sugar grams -		
Total complex grams -		
Total carb calories -		
Total calories of meal -	**cal**	
Total ounces of water with meal -	**ounces**	
Total sodium of meal -	**mgs**	

Time of meal 3 (Lunch) - _________

Food eaten- ____

Drink - ________________________

Carbohydrates	**Protein**	**Fat**
Total carb grams -	Total protein grams -	Total fat grams -
Total fiber grams -	Total protein calories -	Total fat calories -
Total sugar grams -		
Total complex grams -		
Total carb calories -		
Total calories of meal -	**cal**	
Total ounces of water with meal -	**ounces**	
Total sodium of meal -	**mgs**	

Time of meal 4 - _________

Food eaten- ____

Drink - ________________________

Carbohydrates	**Protein**	**Fat**
Total carb grams -	Total protein grams -	Total fat grams -
Total fiber grams -	Total protein calories -	Total fat calories -
Total sugar grams -		
Total complex grams -		
Total carb calories -		
Total calories of meal -	**cal**	
Total ounces of water with meal -	**ounces**	
Total sodium of meal -	**mgs**	

Time of meal 5 - _________

Food eaten- ____

Drink - ________________________

Carbohydrates
Total carb grams -
Total fiber grams -
Total sugar grams -
Total complex grams -
Total carb calories -

Protein
Total protein grams -
Total protein calories -

Fat
Total fat grams -
Total fat calories -

Total calories of meal - cal
Total ounces of water with meal - ounces
Total sodium of meal - mgs

Total ounces of water with meals - ounces
Total ounces of water during workout - ounces
Total ounces of water outside meals - ounces
Total ounces of water today - ounces
Total sodium today - mgs

It's crazy how fast things are going for you. One very important variable that is an integral part of 12 Rounds is variety. Although it is important to change your workouts often to avoid a plateau, variety is even more important to stimulate your mind and to keep you on course to a better and stronger you. One thing you can do to keep things interesting is to try working out in a different environment. You can try another gym or workout at a different time so you can meet new people. Either way, throw some spice in there and keep it hot! And get some sleep too you party animal!

Round 7 - Day 6

It's day 6, and that means cardio and core today. I know it's the weekend and your schedule is a lot different today than it is during the week but make sure you eat 1.5-2.5 hours before you exercise, look over your workout so you'll know what to expect, and put that brain in positive mode so you can knock this day out. Let's go get it!

Which Way You Headed?

Write your three goals about your career. For each goal, give an honest assessment of how much you have achieved to this point by giving a percentage. If you have reached any of these goals, go ahead and write another one to replace the ones you've reached.

My three long term goals about my career including my assessment to this point:

Goal 1 - ____

I feel I have reached ______% of this goal

Goal 2 - ____

I feel I have reached ______% of this goal

Goal 3 - ____

I feel I have reached ______% of this goal

Upper Management

This one is a little different today, but it's one of the best things you can ever do. Think of a person you know who could use some encouragement and a little lift in their spirit. It might be someone with whom you work, a friend, family member, or someone you know from the gym who might be having a hard time. Go to that person and encourage them to keep at it and if you want, share with them some of the things you've learned from 12 Rounds. However you do it, go make someone's day better.

Seeing I to Eye

Take 5 minutes today and think about one great thing you have wanted to happen for a long time. Visualize it exactly how you want it to happen and exactly how you'll feel when it does happen. I know you may think this thing is a long shot, but put your mind to work and it will get a lot closer than you think.

Your Workout – See your workout log.

And the Heart Says…

At some point this evening when you are relaxed, take another heart rate and record it here.

Post workout evening HR ______ Time taken __________

Cleaning Your Plate

Is it bad to work out first thing in the morning on an empty stomach?

In my opinion, I think it's one of the worst things you can do to your body. As I mentioned to you earlier in 12 Rounds, by the time you get up in the mornings, it's been 10-12 hours since you have eaten or drank anything. You can definitely get by without eating before you work out, but you're putting your body in a bad position asking it to function on an empty tank. Always eat 1.5-2.5 hours before you workout, and if that's not possible, then eat something light before you work out at the very least.

You Ate What???

How are you doing keeping up with those calorie breakdowns? One thing I say during almost all of my presentations is that improving your health and changing your lifestyle is not easy and the truth be known; it's a daily fight. When it comes down to it, keeping track of what you're eating and making sure you're eating the right things at the right times is definitely a full time job. That's about the best way I know how to describe it. But let me tell you; it's all very much worth it.

Food Journal

Time of meal 1 - _________

Food eaten- ____

Drink - ________________________

Carbohydrates	**Protein**	**Fat**
Total carb grams -	Total protein grams -	Total fat grams -
Total fiber grams -	Total protein calories -	Total fat calories -
Total sugar grams -		
Total complex grams -		
Total carb calories -		

Total calories of meal - cal
Total ounces of water with meal - ounces
Total sodium of meal - mgs

Time of meal 2 - _________

Food eaten- ____

Drink - ________________________

Carbohydrates	**Protein**	**Fat**
Total carb grams -	Total protein grams -	Total fat grams -
Total fiber grams -	Total protein calories -	Total fat calories -
Total sugar grams -		
Total complex grams -		
Total carb calories -		

Total calories of meal - cal
Total ounces of water with meal - ounces
Total sodium of meal - mgs

Time of meal 3 (Lunch) - _________

Food eaten- ____

Drink - ________________________

Carbohydrates	**Protein**	**Fat**
Total carb grams -	Total protein grams -	Total fat grams -
Total fiber grams -	Total protein calories -	Total fat calories -
Total sugar grams -		
Total complex grams -		
Total carb calories -		

Total calories of meal - cal
Total ounces of water with meal - ounces
Total sodium of meal - mgs

Time of meal 4 - _________

Food eaten- ____

Drink - ________________________

Carbohydrates	**Protein**	**Fat**
Total carb grams -	Total protein grams -	Total fat grams -
Total fiber grams -	Total protein calories -	Total fat calories -
Total sugar grams -		
Total complex grams -		
Total carb calories -		

Total calories of meal - cal
Total ounces of water with meal - ounces
Total sodium of meal - mgs

Time of meal 5 - _________

Food eaten- ____

Drink - ________________________

Carbohydrates	**Protein**	**Fat**
Total carb grams -	Total protein grams -	Total fat grams -
Total fiber grams -	Total protein calories -	Total fat calories -
Total sugar grams -		
Total complex grams -		
Total carb calories -		

Total calories of meal - cal
Total ounces of water with meal - ounces
Total sodium of meal - mgs

Total ounces of water with meals - ounces
Total ounces of water during workout - ounces
Total ounces of water outside meals - ounces
Total ounces of water today - ounces
Total sodium today - mgs

We're almost to the end of another round and there's one thing I always want you to remember wherever you are in your life: Always look and think forward to where you want to go, but every now and then stop, turn around, and look at just how far you've come. From where I'm standing, you've come a long way indeed Champ. Enjoy your success and I'll see you tomorrow for Day 7.

Round 7 - Day 7

It's another day off for you; what do you have planned for your day? If it's fun or has anything to do with fishing or hunting, I'm in! I also like water parks, gun ranges, watching football, hearing a good band, and anything to do with animals so if you do any of those things, give me a ring. Enjoy your day my friend and we will kick it off tomorrow for Round 8!

I took this heart rate when I was…____

Day 7 HR ______ Time taken _______

Food Journal

Time of meal 1 - _________

Food eaten- ____

Drink - ________________________

Carbohydrates	**Protein**	**Fat**
Total carb grams -	Total protein grams -	Total fat grams -
Total fiber grams -	Total protein calories -	Total fat calories -
Total sugar grams -		
Total complex grams -		
Total carb calories -		

Total calories of meal - **cal**
Total ounces of water with meal - **ounces**
Total sodium of meal - **mgs**

Time of meal 2 - _________

Food eaten- ____

Drink - ________________________

Carbohydrates	**Protein**	**Fat**
Total carb grams -	Total protein grams -	Total fat grams -
Total fiber grams -	Total protein calories -	Total fat calories -
Total sugar grams -		
Total complex grams -		
Total carb calories -		

Total calories of meal - **cal**
Total ounces of water with meal - **ounces**
Total sodium of meal - **mgs**

Time of meal 3 (Lunch) - _________

Food eaten- ____

Drink - ________________________

Carbohydrates	**Protein**	**Fat**
Total carb grams -	Total protein grams -	Total fat grams -
Total fiber grams -	Total protein calories -	Total fat calories -
Total sugar grams -		
Total complex grams -		
Total carb calories -		

Total calories of meal - **cal**
Total ounces of water with meal - **ounces**
Total sodium of meal - **mgs**

Time of meal 4 - _________

Food eaten- ____

Drink - ________________________

Carbohydrates	**Protein**	**Fat**
Total carb grams -	Total protein grams -	Total fat grams -
Total fiber grams -	Total protein calories -	Total fat calories -
Total sugar grams -		
Total complex grams -		
Total carb calories -		

Total calories of meal - **cal**
Total ounces of water with meal - **ounces**
Total sodium of meal - **mgs**

Time of meal 5 - _________

Food eaten- ____

Drink - ________________________

Carbohydrates	**Protein**	**Fat**
Total carb grams -	Total protein grams -	Total fat grams -
Total fiber grams -	Total protein calories -	Total fat calories -
Total sugar grams -		
Total complex grams -		
Total carb calories -		

Total calories of meal - **cal**
Total ounces of water with meal - **ounces**
Total sodium of meal - **mgs**

Total ounces of water with meals - **ounces**
Total ounces of water outside meals - **ounces**
Total ounces of water today - **ounces**
Total sodium today - **mgs**

Round 8 – The Right "Fit"

Day 1

There you are! How's that body feeling today? Last week was a great week for you but Round 8 will be your best yet! We're going to put some fire behind those goals of yours, tighten up your eating, and motivate you to your best progress yet. 12 Rounds is about teaching you to improve your life on your terms, and the only way to do that is to make sure the methods you use truly fit you as an individual. As you go through the rest of 12 Rounds, keep your sight on exactly what it is you want out of your life, make sure your goals are helping you get to that point, exercise within your abilities, and let 12 Rounds work its magic. It's your 12 Rounds; make it that way.

"Finding the right workout is a lot like finding the perfect pair of jeans; you look everywhere and try on a bunch of different ones until you find the one that fits you just right. And then you wear the heck out of them."

Bobby Whisnand

It Happened Just Like This!

My doc is a great guy and he's funny which makes my doctor visits so much better. One day I got him good, and the conversation went like this: "Hey doc, why don't you make it easy on yourself and give all your patients the exact same medications and treatments? Don't you think it would save you a ton of time?" He responded with a very weird look on his face and said, "What the heck is wrong with you? Why would I ever do that? That would really mess people up." I then asked him if he thought exercise and eating well were just as important and effective as medications at keeping people healthy. He said, "Yes, what are you getting at goofball?" I said, "Then why do you tell all of your patients to do the exact same thing with exercise and eating well instead of giving them a specific plan that fits their needs, abilities, and health issues?" He paused, stared at me for a bit and said, "Okay, you got me. I never thought about it like that but you're right. Now get out of here and go run or lift something."

That One Thing

There's one thing that's absolutely true when it comes to fitness; *what works for one isn't guaranteed to work for another*. The one thing I want you to do today is to make sure you aren't comparing your fitness results to anyone else. There are far too many variables that affect a person's outcome with their fitness program. If you ever get a chance to read my 2nd book, ***A Body To Die For: The Painful Truth about Exercise***, you'll learn how genetics, PEDs (performance enhancing drugs), and other factors can have a very profound effect on a person's results in fitness. Stick to you; it's all that matters anyway.

Seeing I to Eye

Let's see how good you've gotten at visualization. Take 5 minutes today and visualize yourself being a hero. That's right! You can be the one who saves someone from a dangerous situation, the one who scores the winning touchdown or hits the homerun, the person who comes up with a brilliant idea for a marketing slogan, or the one who closes a huge deal at work. Once you have it, write down your heroic visualization here and go see it happen.

My heroic event is...

___

Your Workout – See your workout log for today's workout.

And the Heart Says…

Let's see what your heart is doing outside of your exercise. Tonight when you're about to go to sleep, take a heart rate and record it here.

Pre Sleep HR - ______ Time taken ________

Cleaning Your Plate

What's the difference between saturated and unsaturated fats?

Fats are often thought of as something to be avoided at all costs, but not all fats are bad. In fact, some fat is needed for good health. The key is choosing the right type of fat. Unsaturated fat can benefit your health, while saturated fat can clog your arteries and increase your risk of a heart attack or stroke.

Saturated fats are solid at room temperature, while unsaturated fats are liquid at room temperature. Saturated fat is found mainly in animal foods like dairy products, fatty beef, lamb, pork, chicken with skin, whole milk, cream, butter, cheese and ice cream. Additionally, baked goods and fried foods can be high in saturated fat because they are made with ingredients loaded with saturated fats, such as butter, cream and lard. Remember those processed foods we talked about?

Unsaturated fats are found in plant foods, fish, liquid vegetable oils (but not tropical oils), canola oil, olive oil, peanut oil and sunflower oil. Examples of oily fish – salmon, tuna, mackerel, herring and trout – contain omega-3 fatty acids, while most nuts and seeds contain a type of unsaturated fat called omega-6 fatty acids. Remember talking about these a few weeks back?

You Ate What???

For your first two meals today, figure up the percentage of carbohydrates, proteins, and fats. Here's how you do it:

You already have the total calories for each type of nutrition so all you have to do is divide the number of calories for each type of nutrition by the total number of calories for the entire meal. This is what it looks like:

- Total carbohydrate calories = 200
- Total calories for the entire meal = 600
- 200/600 = 33.3 which means 33.3 % of your meal was carbs.

Food Journal

Time of meal 1 - _________

Food eaten- ____

Drink - ________________________

Carbohydrates	**Protein**	**Fat**
Total crab grams -	Total protein grams -	Total fat grams -
Total fiber grams -	Total protein calories -	Total fat calories
Total sugar grams -		Total saturated
Total complex grams -		Total unsaturated -
Total carb calories -		
Percentage of meal - %	Percentage of meal - %	Percentage of meal - %

Total calories of meal - cal
Total ounces of water with meal - ounces
Total sodium of meal - mgs

Time of meal 2 - _________

Food eaten- ____

Drink - ________________________

Carbohydrates	**Protein**	**Fat**
Total crab grams -	Total protein grams -	Total fat grams -
Total fiber grams -	Total protein calories -	Total fat calories
Total sugar grams -		Total saturated
Total complex grams -		Total unsaturated -
Total carb calories -		
Percentage of meal - %	Percentage of meal - %	Percentage of meal - %

Total calories of meal - cal
Total ounces of water with meal - ounces
Total sodium of meal - mgs

Time of meal 3 (Lunch) - _________

Food eaten- ____

Drink - ________________________

Carbohydrates	**Protein**	**Fat**
Total crab grams -	Total protein grams -	Total fat grams -
Total fiber grams -	Total protein calories -	Total fat calories
Total sugar grams -		Total saturated
Total complex grams -		Total unsaturated -
Total carb calories -		

Total calories of meal - cal
Total ounces of water with meal - ounces
Total sodium of meal - mgs

Time of meal 4 - _________

Food eaten- ____

Drink - ________________________

Carbohydrates	**Protein**	**Fat**
Total crab grams -	Total protein grams -	Total fat grams -
Total fiber grams -	Total protein calories -	Total fat calories
Total sugar grams -		Total saturated
Total complex grams -		Total unsaturated -
Total carb calories -		

Total calories of meal - cal
Total ounces of water with meal - ounces
Total sodium of meal - mgs

Time of meal 5 - _________

Food eaten- ____

Drink - ________________________

Carbohydrates	**Protein**	**Fat**
Total crab grams -	Total protein grams -	Total fat grams -
Total fiber grams -	Total protein calories -	Total fat calories
Total sugar grams -		Total saturated
Total complex grams -		Total unsaturated -
Total carb calories -		

Total calories of meal - cal
Total ounces of water with meal - ounces
Total sodium of meal - mgs

Total ounces of water with meals - ounces
Total ounces of water during workout - ounces
Total ounces of water outside meals - ounces
Total ounces of water today - ounces
Total sodium today - mgs

You are kicking butt! We ramped it up a little today but you made it look easy. Think back to your first day on Round 1; a lot has changed hasn't it? Keep it up; you've got something very good going on. I'll see you tomorrow.

Round 8 - Day 2

It's day 2 and that means core and cardio today. I have a question for you: What things do you think about during your workouts? Whatever it is, make sure they are positive things and no matter how hard it is sometimes, if a negative or stressful thought tries to come sneaking in during your workouts, cut if off and replace it with something good. Remember; where the head goes, the body follows and you my friend are always in control of what gets in that head of yours.

Which Way You Headed?

Write your three goals about things other than fitness. Below each one, write one thing you can do **this week** to help you reach each goal.

Goal 1 - ____

One thing I can do this week to help me reach this goal is…

____

Goal 2 - ____

One thing I can do this week to help me reach this goal is…

____

Goal 3 - ____

One thing I can do this week to help me reach this goal is…

____

Seeing I to Eye

Think of a long term goal you had before you started 12 Rounds. It might be a weight loss goal, a financial goal, something to do with your relationship, your home, paying off credit card bills, or anything else. Just make sure you had it before you started 12 Rounds and it's not one of your current goals. Once you have it, write it down here and visualize yourself reaching that long awaited goal.

One long term goal I had before I started 12 Rounds is…

____

Upper Management

One of the biggest reasons many people do not exercise is their time and schedule. They might have the best intentions but one unexpected thing happens and the whole plan is blown up. I'm going to give you two things you can do to make sure you make your exercise appointment every single time.

- Schedule and treat all exercise sessions just like a work appointment or anything else which you cannot miss.
- If the weekdays are very hectic for you or you have an unpredictable work schedule, start each round of 12 Rounds on a Friday. This means you get three of your five workouts done on the weekend leaving only two to get done during the week. I know it takes time from your weekend but you have to make those workouts a priority.

Your Workout – See your workout log for today's workout.

Cleaning Your Plate

What are antioxidants and should you take them?

Antioxidants are substances that may protect cells in your body from free radical damage that can occur from exposure to certain chemicals, smoking, pollution, radiation, and as a byproduct of normal metabolism. Dietary antioxidants include selenium, vitamin A and related carotenoids, vitamins C and E, plus various phytochemicals such as lycopene, lutein, and quercetin. Consuming foods rich in antioxidants may be good for your heart health and may also help to lower your risk of infections and some forms of cancer.

You can get antioxidants in supplement form or you can get them from foods such as fruits, vegetables, nuts, and whole grains and smaller amounts of antioxidants in meats, poultry and fish.

Now, should you take an antioxidant supplement?

I think it's a good idea and I encourage all of my clients to take one called Astaxanthin. This is a very powerful antioxidant which is even more powerful than blueberries; look it up.

You Ate What???

Remember to figure up the percentage of carbs, protein, and fat for your first two meals today. While you're at it, take a real close look at the amount of calories you're eating with each meal and total calories for the day.

Food Journal

Time of meal 1 - _________

Food eaten- ____

Drink - ________________________

Carbohydrates		**Protein**		**Fat**	
Total crab grams -		Total protein grams -		Total fat grams -	
Total fiber grams -		Total protein calories -		Total fat calories	
Total sugar grams -				Total saturated	
Total complex grams -				Total unsaturated -	
Total carb calories -					
Percentage of meal -	%	Percentage of meal -	%	Percentage of meal -	%
Total calories of meal -		**cal**			
Total ounces of water with meal -		**ounces**			
Total sodium of meal -		**mgs**			

Time of meal 2 - _________

Food eaten- ____

Drink - ________________________

Carbohydrates	**Protein**	**Fat**
Total crab grams -	Total protein grams -	Total fat grams -
Total fiber grams -	Total protein calories -	Total fat calories
Total sugar grams -		Total saturated
Total complex grams -		Total unsaturated -
Total carb calories -		
Percentage of meal - %	Percentage of meal - %	Percentage of meal - %

Total calories of meal - cal
Total ounces of water with meal - ounces
Total sodium of meal - mgs

Time of meal 3 (Lunch) - _________

Food eaten- ____

Drink - ________________________

Carbohydrates	**Protein**	**Fat**
Total crab grams -	Total protein grams -	Total fat grams -
Total fiber grams -	Total protein calories -	Total fat calories
Total sugar grams -		Total saturated
Total complex grams -		Total unsaturated -
Total carb calories -		

Total calories of meal - cal
Total ounces of water with meal - ounces
Total sodium of meal - mgs

Time of meal 4 - _________

Food eaten- ____

Drink - ________________________

Carbohydrates	**Protein**	**Fat**
Total crab grams -	Total protein grams -	Total fat grams -
Total fiber grams -	Total protein calories -	Total fat calories
Total sugar grams -		Total saturated
Total complex grams -		Total unsaturated -
Total carb calories -		

Total calories of meal - cal
Total ounces of water with meal - ounces
Total sodium of meal - mgs

Time of meal 5 - _________

Food eaten- ____

Drink - ________________________

Carbohydrates	**Protein**	**Fat**
Total crab grams -	Total protein grams -	Total fat grams -
Total fiber grams -	Total protein calories -	Total fat calories
Total sugar grams -		Total saturated
Total complex grams -		Total unsaturated -
Total carb calories -		

Total calories of meal - cal
Total ounces of water with meal - ounces
Total sodium of meal - mgs

Total ounces of water with meals - ounces
Total ounces of water during workout - ounces
Total ounces of water outside meals - ounces
Total ounces of water today - ounces
Total sodium today - mgs

And The Heart Says…
At some point in the middle of your day, take a heart rate and record it here.

Afternoon HR-________ Time taken - _______

How about that new core routine you did today? Those planks and one leg bridges can really do a number on your core. I'm sure you did awesome and now it's time to recuperate, relax, eat some good food, and look over your workout coming up tomorrow. Get ready for a great leg day!

Round 8 – Day 3

Is it hump day today? Nope; it's LEG DAY! You'll be doing a unilateral reverse leg workout, so make sure you get your workout log filled out and ready to go and I'll see you in the gym. Oh yeah; don't forget to drink plenty of water before you workout.

That One Thing

I'm going to throw you a curve today. Where's that list I asked you to print out? Do you have it where you can see it every day? I'm going to assume you printed it out and it's right in front of you at least a couple of times a day. Okay, your one thing to do today is to pick another thing on that list, write it down here, and make a plan to get it done by the end of this week.

One more thing on my list I'm going to get done this week is…

___

Seeing I to Eye

Are you ready to travel back in time? Go to that secluded place of yours, completely clear your mind of all distractions, and spend 5 minutes today visualizing yourself as you were 20 years ago. Once you can see your younger self, visualize having more energy, being stronger, and having less stress. If you are younger than 40, go back 10 years and visualize the same things. Okay youngster; go to it.

Your Workout – See your workout log for today's workout.

And the Heart Says…

While you're at work today and sitting at your desk, take a heart rate and write it down here. Make sure you've been sitting for at least 5 minutes before you take it.

Resting HR - ______ Time Taken - ________

Cleaning Your Plate

Is there really such a thing as a fat burner?

This is a tough one because there are tons of people who swear by them yet there are no conclusive studies that say they truly work. What exactly are people using as "fat burners" these days? Fat burners are essentially pills which contain certain herbal ingredients such as Ephedra, HCA, Chitosan and Pyruvate, all of which claim to either increase energy, stimulate your metabolism and/or suppress your appetite.

Now, do fat burners work?

It's hard to say. Try to find a conclusive study about any dietary supplement, including so-called fat burners, and you're in for a long day. What we do know is that most supplements need further study, and more importantly, the purity of supplements is definitely suspect. Supplements aren't standardized so you don't know if what's listed on the bottle is what you're getting. Plus, no one knows what the long-term effects of these supplements are and, even scarier, how they interact with other medications. My advice to you on fat burners or any supplement for that matter: Be careful! If you're dead set on taking any supplement, do your diligence and research it first, keep a journal on the effects or lack of, and use them in moderation. If you take any kind of mediation, check with your doctor before you take anything. Do we have a deal?

You Ate What???

For now, keep everything the same. Take a close look at those percentages of carbs, proteins, and fats for two meals but start alternating which two meals you track. A good ratio for you to shoot for at this point in the game is 40% carbs, 30% protein, and 30% fats. Starting next week, I'm going to show you how to manipulate these percentages according to your body weight goals.

Food Journal

Time of meal 1 - _________

Food eaten- ____

Drink - ________________________

Carbohydrates	**Protein**	**Fat**
Total crab grams -	Total protein grams -	Total fat grams -
Total fiber grams -	Total protein calories -	Total fat calories
Total sugar grams -		Total saturated
Total complex grams -		Total unsaturated -
Total carb calories -		
Percentage of meal - %	Percentage of meal - %	Percentage of meal - %

Total calories of meal - **cal**
Total ounces of water with meal - **ounces**
Total sodium of meal - **mgs**

Time of meal 2 - _________

Food eaten- ____

Drink - ________________________

Carbohydrates	**Protein**	**Fat**
Total crab grams -	Total protein grams -	Total fat grams -
Total fiber grams -	Total protein calories -	Total fat calories
Total sugar grams -		Total saturated
Total complex grams -		Total unsaturated -
Total carb calories -		

Total calories of meal - **cal**
Total ounces of water with meal - **ounces**
Total sodium of meal - **mgs**

Time of meal 3 (Lunch) - _________

Food eaten- ____

Drink - ________________________

Carbohydrates	**Protein**	**Fat**
Total crab grams -	Total protein grams -	Total fat grams -
Total fiber grams -	Total protein calories -	Total fat calories
Total sugar grams -		Total saturated
Total complex grams -		Total unsaturated -
Total carb calories -		

Total calories of meal - **cal**
Total ounces of water with meal - **ounces**
Total sodium of meal - **mgs**

Time of meal 4 - _________

Food eaten- ____

Drink - ________________________

Carbohydrates	**Protein**	**Fat**
Total crab grams -	Total protein grams -	Total fat grams -
Total fiber grams -	Total protein calories -	Total fat calories
Total sugar grams -		Total saturated
Total complex grams -		Total unsaturated -
Total carb calories -		

Total calories of meal - **cal**
Total ounces of water with meal - **ounces**
Total sodium of meal - **mgs**

Time of meal 5 - _________

Food eaten- ____

Drink - ________________________

Carbohydrates	**Protein**	**Fat**
Total crab grams -	Total protein grams -	Total fat grams -
Total fiber grams -	Total protein calories -	Total fat calories
Total sugar grams -		Total saturated
Total complex grams -		Total unsaturated -
Total carb calories -		

Total calories of meal - **cal**
Total ounces of water with meal - **ounces**
Total sodium of meal - **mgs**

Total ounces of water with meals - **ounces**
Total ounces of water during workout - **ounces**
Total ounces of water outside meals - **ounces**
Total ounces of water today - **ounces**
Total sodium today - **mgs**

You're going to be a master chemist by the time I get done with you; a master chemist who's in darn good shape. Great job today on everything: Your workout, your goals, your positive outlook, and of course your unbelievably detailed food journal. Now all that's left is to relax, enjoy your evening, lock down on some good sleep, and dream of something awesome happening to you.

Round 8 - Day 4

How are those legs feeling this morning? A good thing for you to do is to start taking note of the level of soreness you're having the day after your workouts. If your soreness is severe and lasting for more than 72 hours, it's time to back off and reduce your workouts. It's Day 4 and you know what's up: A day off for you. Let's see what else I have for you to do.

"Knowing what works for you is the start of knowing what won't work for others."

Bobby Whisnand

It Happened Just Like This!

I was presenting to a group of personal trainers and one question I asked them was, "What do you guys think are the most neglected parts of exercise programs other than not eating right and not using good form and technique?" Their two most common answers were… not doing enough cardio and not warming up. I then said "although these are things that are neglected a lot, they aren't the most neglected. The most neglected parts of many exercise programs out there are not keeping a detailed workout log and not keeping a food journal. I then told them that the best advice I could ever give them was this: Never assume anything about any client, design their workout program around their individual needs, never give them a generic program, journal every single thing they do including heart rates, and have them keep a food journal and review it once a week with them.

Individualized fitness is a very rare thing; most people just do what everyone else is doing and hope for the best. With 12 Rounds, you're learning to do the things that work best for you, and that food journal you're keeping; priceless!

Which Way You Headed?

Write your three goals about your fitness. Below each one, write one thing you can do **this week t**o help you reach each goal.

Goal 1 - ____

One thing I can do this week to help me reach this goal is…

____

Goal 2 - ____

One thing I can do this week to help me reach this goal is…

____

Goal 3 - ____

One thing I can do this week to help me reach this goal is…

____

Seeing I to Eye

Isn't it amazing how you can remember something funny from 10, 20, even 30 or more years ago? Think back to a very funny event in your life and take 5 minutes today and relive it a few times. I won't make you write this one down because if your funny memories are anywhere close to what mine are, you might get in trouble if someone reads it. Go ahead; have a good laugh today.

Upper Management

A Time for Change

If there is a part of your life where you are unhappy, don't be afraid to make a change. Sometimes we end up in places where we never intended to be; maybe it's a bad relationship, a career choice, a financial mistake, being unhealthy, or many other circumstances that greatly strain our ability to be happy. The best advice I can give you is to not wait on things to get better and start making changes for yourself. As hard as it is sometimes, you can never let anyone else determine how you live. Stand up, be strong, and get moving to a better and happier life.

No Workout Today! - Pizza? Who said pizza? Maybe for one of your cheat meals, right?

And the Heart Says…

Take at least one heart rate today whenever you want. Just make sure you write down when and under what circumstances you took it.

Today I took my heart rate when I was… ____

Day 4 HR - ______ Time taken - ________

Cleaning Your Plate

One of the biggest deterrents to eating well is travel. If you travel for work you know exactly what I mean, right? Here are some tips to help you stay on your eating plan when you're on the road.

- Do some research on healthy restaurants and other places to eat before you travel.
- If it's a long stay, get a hotel room with a kitchen or at least a refrigerator so you can cook your own food or keep good food in your room and avoid restaurants.
- If you have no other choice than to eat at restaurants, eat at the ones where you can order healthy foods.
- When you order your food at restaurants, tell them no bread or chips prior to your meal, order your food with sauce on the side, and ask them to bake or steam your food instead of grilling it in oil or frying it.
- Avoid fast foods at all cost.

You Ate What???

I know these food journals take some time but it's well worth it to help you get exactly where you want to go. Think about it like this: Your body listens to everything you say and one of the most common ways to communicate with it is by what you eat and drink. If you want your body to look, act, and feel a certain way, you have to tell it exactly how to do so by what you eat and drink. And keeping track of what goes in that body is the only way to do it right.

Food Journal

Time of meal 1 - _________

Food eaten- ____

Drink - ________________________

Carbohydrates		**Protein**		**Fat**	
Total crab grams -		Total protein grams -		Total fat grams -	
Total fiber grams -		Total protein calories -		Total fat calories	
Total sugar grams -				Total saturated	
Total complex grams -				Total unsaturated -	
Total carb calories -					
Percentage of meal -	%	Percentage of meal -	%	Percentage of meal -	%

Total calories of meal - **cal**
Total ounces of water with meal - **ounces**
Total sodium of meal - **mgs**

Time of meal 2 - _________

Food eaten- ____

Drink - ________________________

Carbohydrates		**Protein**		**Fat**	
Total crab grams -		Total protein grams -		Total fat grams -	
Total fiber grams -		Total protein calories -		Total fat calories	
Total sugar grams -				Total saturated	
Total complex grams -				Total unsaturated -	
Total carb calories -					
Percentage of meal -	%	Percentage of meal -	%	Percentage of meal -	%

Total calories of meal - **cal**
Total ounces of water with meal - **ounces**
Total sodium of meal - **mgs**

Time of meal 3 (Lunch) - _________

Food eaten- ____

Drink - ________________________

Carbohydrates	**Protein**	**Fat**
Total crab grams -	Total protein grams -	Total fat grams -
Total fiber grams -	Total protein calories -	Total fat calories
Total sugar grams -		Total saturated
Total complex grams -		Total unsaturated -
Total carb calories -		

Total calories of meal - **cal**
Total ounces of water with meal - **ounces**
Total sodium of meal - **mgs**

Time of meal 4 - _________

Food eaten- ____

Drink - ________________________

Carbohydrates	**Protein**	**Fat**
Total crab grams -	Total protein grams -	Total fat grams -
Total fiber grams -	Total protein calories -	Total fat calories
Total sugar grams -		Total saturated
Total complex grams -		Total unsaturated -
Total carb calories -		

Total calories of meal - cal
Total ounces of water with meal - ounces
Total sodium of meal - mgs

Time of meal 5 - _________

Food eaten- ____

Drink - ________________________

Carbohydrates	**Protein**	**Fat**
Total crab grams -	Total protein grams -	Total fat grams -
Total fiber grams -	Total protein calories -	Total fat calories
Total sugar grams -		Total saturated
Total complex grams -		Total unsaturated -
Total carb calories -		

Total calories of meal - cal
Total ounces of water with meal - ounces
Total sodium of meal - mgs

Total ounces of water with meals - ounces
Total ounces of water outside meals - ounces
Total ounces of water today - ounces
Total sodium today - mgs

Way to go Champ! Every single day of 12 Rounds you complete is another big step to being exactly where you want to be. Stay strong, stay positive, feed and rest that body, and we will knock Day 5 straight out.

Round 8 - Day 5

Time to work those guns! It's back and bicep day again; are you ready for it? Let's go find out.

That One Thing

Think about your food journal for a moment. What do you think is the biggest change you have made with your eating to this point with 12 Rounds. Once you got it, write it down here.

The biggest change I have made with my eating from doing 12 Rounds is...

____

Seeing I to Eye

Think about the biggest award you would like to receive and take 5 minutes today and see yourself getting that award. It could be top salesperson, getting a higher degree of education, or even shoot for the stars and go for something like a Nobel Prize, man or women of the year, athlete of the year, or whatever you want. Once you decide what award you're about to receive, write it down here and go get that thing!

The absolute biggest award I'm about to see myself receive is...

____

Your Workout – See your workout log .

And the Heart Says...

Sometime tonight after dinner and when you have been relaxing for about an hour, take and record a heart rate.

Evening resting HR ______ Time taken ______

Cleaning Your Plate

If you miss a meal during your day, should you make up the calories with another meal?

This can get tricky so you have to careful here. It really depends on which meal you miss. If you miss breakfast, I would increase the amount I eat during meal 2. If you miss lunch, I would make up the calories during meal 4. If you miss dinner, you can eat later before you go to bed but I would only eat protein and green vegetables unless you're trying to gain weight. In that case, I'd eat the full meal.

If you miss one of your snacks like in meal 2 and 4, I would only make up about half the calories during lunch or dinner; you don't want to eat too much at once.

Try not to miss any meals but if you do, make it up like I show you above and don't worry about it.

You Ate What???

I know it's been a few days since I brought this up, but keep on evaluating your meals and start replacing the bad foods with healthier choices. Also, keep figuring those percentages of carbs, proteins and fats for two meals a day and see how close you are to the 40/30/30 ratio. If you are trying to lose weight, start reducing your calories across each meal, but just a little at a time.

Food Journal

Time of meal 1 - __________

Food eaten- ____

Drink - ____________________

Carbohydrates	**Protein**	**Fat**
Total crab grams -	Total protein grams -	Total fat grams -
Total fiber grams -	Total protein calories -	Total fat calories
Total sugar grams -		Total saturated
Total complex grams -		Total unsaturated -
Total carb calories -		
Percentage of meal - %	Percentage of meal - %	Percentage of meal - %

Total calories of meal - cal
Total ounces of water with meal - ounces
Total sodium of meal - mgs

Time of meal 2 - _________

Food eaten- ____

Drink - ________________________

Carbohydrates	**Protein**	**Fat**
Total crab grams -	Total protein grams -	Total fat grams -
Total fiber grams -	Total protein calories -	Total fat calories
Total sugar grams -		Total saturated
Total complex grams -		Total unsaturated -
Total carb calories -		
Percentage of meal - %	Percentage of meal - %	Percentage of meal - %

Total calories of meal - cal
Total ounces of water with meal - ounces
Total sodium of meal - mgs

Time of meal 3 (Lunch) - _________

Food eaten- ____

Drink - ________________________

Carbohydrates	**Protein**	**Fat**
Total crab grams -	Total protein grams -	Total fat grams -
Total fiber grams -	Total protein calories -	Total fat calories
Total sugar grams -		Total saturated
Total complex grams -		Total unsaturated -
Total carb calories -		

Total calories of meal - cal
Total ounces of water with meal - ounces
Total sodium of meal - mgs

Time of meal 4 - _________

Food eaten- ____

Drink - ________________________

Carbohydrates	**Protein**	**Fat**
Total crab grams -	Total protein grams -	Total fat grams -
Total fiber grams -	Total protein calories -	Total fat calories
Total sugar grams -		Total saturated
Total complex grams -		Total unsaturated -
Total carb calories -		

Total calories of meal - **cal**
Total ounces of water with meal - **ounces**
Total sodium of meal - **mgs**

Time of meal 5 - _________

Food eaten- ____

Drink - ________________________

Carbohydrates	**Protein**	**Fat**
Total crab grams -	Total protein grams -	Total fat grams -
Total fiber grams -	Total protein calories -	Total fat calories
Total sugar grams -		Total saturated
Total complex grams -		Total unsaturated -
Total carb calories -		

Total calories of meal - **cal**
Total ounces of water with meal - **ounces**
Total sodium of meal - **mgs**

Total ounces of water with meals - **ounces**
Total ounces of water during workout - **ounces**
Total ounces of water outside meals - **ounces**
Total ounces of water today - **ounces**
Total sodium today - **mgs**

How do you feel you did today? Did you feel good during your back and bicep workout? If you are running low on energy during and after your workouts, start paying close attention to what and when you're eating. To help you with this, next week I'm going to start showing you how to manipulate your diet to make sure you're getting the right kinds of nutrition to fit your needs. Now go get some good food and if you have some left over, send it to me.

Round 8 - Day 6

We're going to really mix it up today for your core and cardio workout. I'm going to combine all of it for one big circuit so get ready to sweat and burn.

Which Way You Headed?

Write your three goals about your career. Below each one, write one thing you can do **this week t**o help you reach each goal.

Goal 1 - ____

One thing I can do this week to help me reach this goal is…

____

Goal 2 - ____

One thing I can do this week to help me reach this goal is…

____

Goal 3 - ____

One thing I can do this week to help me reach this goal is…

____

Upper Management

Okay, it's time to get another set of eyes and ears on your goals. Get with the person with whom you are sharing your goals and go over all nine goals. Show them the "Which Way You Headed" sections in this round so they can see all of your goals and make notes here as well if you want. This is a great time for you to reflect on just how far you've come.

Seeing I to Eye

Are you ready for a challenge? Take all the time you need today to do this but make sure it's in a secluded place with no distractions. Pick three of your long term goals and visualize yourself reaching all three of them, one at a time. Make sure you include as many senses as you can like sound, feelings, colors, and of course seeing. Make yourself proud today!

Your Workout – See your workout log for today's workout.

And the Heart Says…

At some point this evening when you are relaxed, take another heart rate and record it here.

Post workout evening HR ______ Time taken ______ ___

Cleaning Your Plate

Is it okay to eat bread?

Absolutely it is! Bread is just like any other food; you have to be careful of how much you eat, when you eat it, make sure it's whole, natural, and unrefined, and keep track of when you eat it. You definitely want to stay away from the refined white breads, but whole unprocessed wheat bread is not only okay to eat, it's very nutritious. Just be sure to limit how much you eat and if losing weight is your goal, limit how much bread you eat just like you do any of your other complex carbs.

You Ate What???

Between today and tomorrow night, look back through your food journals and see how well you're doing. If you aren't filling your food journal out completely, make an effort this next week to make it complete.

Food Journal

Time of meal 1 - _________

Food eaten- ____

Drink - ________________________

Carbohydrates	**Protein**	**Fat**
Total crab grams -	Total protein grams -	Total fat grams -
Total fiber grams -	Total protein calories -	Total fat calories
Total sugar grams -		Total saturated
Total complex grams -		Total unsaturated -
Total carb calories -		
Percentage of meal - %	Percentage of meal - %	Percentage of meal - %

Total calories of meal - **cal**
Total ounces of water with meal - **ounces**
Total sodium of meal - **mgs**

Time of meal 2 - _________

Food eaten- ____

Drink - ________________________

Carbohydrates	**Protein**	**Fat**
Total crab grams -	Total protein grams -	Total fat grams -
Total fiber grams -	Total protein calories -	Total fat calories
Total sugar grams -		Total saturated
Total complex grams -		Total unsaturated -
Total carb calories -		
Percentage of meal - %	Percentage of meal - %	Percentage of meal - %

Total calories of meal - **cal**
Total ounces of water with meal - **ounces**
Total sodium of meal - **mgs**

Time of meal 3 (Lunch) - _________

Food eaten- ____

Drink - ________________________

Carbohydrates	**Protein**	**Fat**
Total crab grams -	Total protein grams -	Total fat grams -
Total fiber grams -	Total protein calories -	Total fat calories
Total sugar grams -		Total saturated
Total complex grams -		Total unsaturated -
Total carb calories -		

Total calories of meal - **cal**
Total ounces of water with meal - **ounces**
Total sodium of meal - **mgs**

Time of meal 4 - _________

Food eaten- ____

Drink - ________________________

Carbohydrates
Total crab grams -
Total fiber grams -
Total sugar grams -
Total complex grams -
Total carb calories -

Protein
Total protein grams -
Total protein calories -

Fat
Total fat grams -
Total fat calories
Total saturated
Total unsaturated -

Total calories of meal - cal
Total ounces of water with meal - ounces
Total sodium of meal - mgs

Time of meal 5 - _________

Food eaten- ____

Drink - ________________________

Carbohydrates
Total crab grams -
Total fiber grams -
Total sugar grams -
Total complex grams -
Total carb calories -

Protein
Total protein grams -
Total protein calories -

Fat
Total fat grams -
Total fat calories
Total saturated
Total unsaturated -

Total calories of meal - cal
Total ounces of water with meal - ounces
Total sodium of meal - mgs

Total ounces of water with meals - ounces
Total ounces of water during workout - ounces
Total ounces of water outside meals - ounces
Total ounces of water today - ounces
Total sodium today - mgs

One more day and Round 8 is in the books. Keep thinking good things and good things will happen to you; they're happening right now!

Round 8 - Day 7

What kind of things are you doing on your days off from exercise? Whatever they are, enjoy yourself and don't forget to invite me every now and then; I might eat all of your food and embarrass you, but it will be a blast.

I took this heart rate when I was…____

Day 7 HR ______ Time taken _______

Food Journal

Time of meal 1 - _________

Food eaten- ____

Drink - ________________________

Carbohydrates		**Protein**		**Fat**	
Total crab grams -		Total protein grams -		Total fat grams -	
Total fiber grams -		Total protein calories -		Total fat calories	
Total sugar grams -				Total saturated	
Total complex grams -				Total unsaturated -	
Total carb calories -					
Percentage of meal -	%	Percentage of meal -	%	Percentage of meal -	%

Total calories of meal - **cal**
Total ounces of water with meal - **ounces**
Total sodium of meal - **mgs**

Time of meal 2 - _________

Food eaten- ____

Drink - ________________________

Carbohydrates		**Protein**		**Fat**	
Total crab grams -		Total protein grams -		Total fat grams -	
Total fiber grams -		Total protein calories -		Total fat calories	
Total sugar grams -				Total saturated	
Total complex grams -				Total unsaturated -	
Total carb calories -					
Percentage of meal -	%	Percentage of meal -	%	Percentage of meal -	%

Total calories of meal - **cal**
Total ounces of water with meal - **ounces**
Total sodium of meal - **mgs**

Time of meal 3 (Lunch) - _________

Food eaten- ____

Drink - ________________________

Carbohydrates	**Protein**	**Fat**
Total crab grams -	Total protein grams -	Total fat grams -
Total fiber grams -	Total protein calories -	Total fat calories
Total sugar grams -		Total saturated
Total complex grams -		Total unsaturated -
Total carb calories -		

Total calories of meal - **cal**
Total ounces of water with meal - **ounces**
Total sodium of meal - **mgs**

Time of meal 4 - _________

Food eaten- ____

Drink - ________________________

Carbohydrates	**Protein**	**Fat**
Total crab grams -	Total protein grams -	Total fat grams -
Total fiber grams -	Total protein calories -	Total fat calories
Total sugar grams -		Total saturated
Total complex grams -		Total unsaturated -
Total carb calories -		

Total calories of meal - **cal**
Total ounces of water with meal - **ounces**
Total sodium of meal - **mgs**

Time of meal 5 - _________

Food eaten- ____

Drink - ________________________

Carbohydrates	**Protein**	**Fat**
Total crab grams -	Total protein grams -	Total fat grams -
Total fiber grams -	Total protein calories -	Total fat calories
Total sugar grams -		Total saturated
Total complex grams -		Total unsaturated -
Total carb calories -		

Total calories of meal - **cal**
Total ounces of water with meal - **ounces**
Total sodium of meal - **mgs**

Total ounces of water with meals - **ounces**
Total ounces of water during workout - **ounces**
Total ounces of water outside meals - **ounces**
Total ounces of water today - **ounces**
Total sodium today - **mgs**

Round 9 – Breaking Barriers

Day 1

I've decided to raise the stakes with 12 Rounds and get you out of your comfort zone this week. Variety is the spice of life, right? I know you're doing great so far but I want more for you so let's kick it off and have the best round yet!

"Being comfortable is okay and kind of average, but being tenacious, inspired, and unsatisfied is where all the fun stuff happens." Bobby Whisnand

It Happened Just Like This!

A few years ago, I met a new friend, and it was obvious he was not confident or comfortable around women. He loved to go out but he did the same thing every single time; he stood with his arms crossed, kept his head down, and wouldn't say a word when a girl would walk by. One day I brought it up and he said, "I just feel like they're going to think I'm stupid and they're not going to like me." I said, "You're wrong buddy, they won't think that at all and I can prove it." Two nights later we went out and I could see he was terrified. I told him that for every girl I went up to and introduced myself, he had to do the same with another girl. That's all he had to do; just walk up, say hi, tell her to have a nice night and walk off. The first two or three were very shaky but about half way through the night, he was doing a lot more than saying hello. He was having lengthy conversations, having drinks (buying them mainly), and he even got two phone numbers to top it all off. Man was he feeling good! By the way, his comfort level with women wasn't the only thing that got better; soon after that he volunteered for a huge work project that required a lot of speaking and presenting to large groups of people, and he did so well that he was promoted twice in one year. New man, new confidence, new life!

Get out of your comfort zone; there's a whole new world for you to see.

That One Thing

What is one big thing you've always wanted to do but you haven't done it yet because you're too embarrassed, shy, or you just don't think you can do it?

Write it down here:

____

Seeing I to Eye

You just wrote down one thing you've always wanted to do but you're too shy or too uncomfortable to actually do it. Take 5-6 minutes today in that quiet place and see yourself doing it exactly how you want to.

Your Workout – See your workout log .

And the Heart Says…

Tonight when you're about to go to sleep, take a heart rate and record it here. Coming up next week, we're going to start looking back at all of these heart rates you've taken and see what's happening.

Pre Sleep HR - ______ Time taken ________

Cleaning Your Plate

What exactly are high energy foods?

There are actually two kinds of high energy foods; those that give you quick energy and those that give you sustained energy. Quick energy foods are the ones that have natural simple sugar in them like fruits. If you remember, simple sugars are broken down very quickly by your body and therefore are available as quick high energy. The only problem is the energy from simple sugars is very short lived, so this is where timing comes into play. Eating fruit throughout your day is a great idea and can give you a quick boost in energy, but at all cost stay away from those processed simple sugars found in many foods today.

The other type of high energy food is from foods high in complex carbohydrates like whole grains, starchy vegetables, and nuts. These complex carbohydrate foods provide high energy but also provide sustained energy. Complex carbohydrates take anywhere from 1-2 hours for your body to break them down for energy, but once this breakdown happens, it provides high long lasting energy for your body. This is exactly why I tell you throughout 12 Rounds to always eat 1.5-2.5 hours before you workout as well as to greatly reduce or eliminate complex carbs from your meal late at night.

You Ate What???

Let's take a few more days figuring up these percentages and then I'll start showing you how to make changes to fit your body weight goals.

Here's that formula again in case you forgot. Use this same formula for protein and fats.

- Total carbohydrate calories = 200
- Total calories for the entire meal = 600
- 200/600 = 33.3 which means 33.3 % of your meal was carbs.

Food Journal

Time of meal 1 - _________

Food eaten- ____

Drink - ________________________

Carbohydrates	**Protein**	**Fat**
Total crab grams -	Total protein grams -	Total fat grams -
Total fiber grams -	Total protein calories -	Total fat calories
Total sugar grams -		Total saturated
Total complex grams -		Total unsaturated -
Total carb calories -		
Percentage of meal - %	Percentage of meal - %	Percentage of meal - %

Total calories of meal - cal
Total ounces of water with meal - ounces
Total sodium of meal - mgs

Time of meal 2 - _________

Food eaten- ____

Drink - ________________________

Carbohydrates		**Protein**		**Fat**	
Total crab grams -		Total protein grams -		Total fat grams -	
Total fiber grams -		Total protein calories -		Total fat calories	
Total sugar grams -				Total saturated	
Total complex grams -				Total unsaturated -	
Total carb calories -					
Percentage of meal -	%	Percentage of meal -	%	Percentage of meal -	%
Total calories of meal -		**cal**			
Total ounces of water with meal -		**ounces**			
Total sodium of meal -		**mgs**			

Time of meal 3 (Lunch) - _________

Food eaten- ____

Drink - ________________________

Carbohydrates	**Protein**	**Fat**
Total crab grams -	Total protein grams -	Total fat grams -
Total fiber grams -	Total protein calories -	Total fat calories
Total sugar grams -		Total saturated
Total complex grams -		Total unsaturated -
Total carb calories -		
Total calories of meal -	**cal**	
Total ounces of water with meal -	**ounces**	
Total sodium of meal -	**mgs**	

Time of meal 4 - _________

Food eaten- ____

Drink - ________________________

Carbohydrates	**Protein**	**Fat**
Total crab grams -	Total protein grams -	Total fat grams -
Total fiber grams -	Total protein calories -	Total fat calories
Total sugar grams -		Total saturated
Total complex grams -		Total unsaturated -
Total carb calories -		
Total calories of meal -	**cal**	
Total ounces of water with meal -	**ounces**	
Total sodium of meal -	**mgs**	

Time of meal 5 - ________

Food eaten- ____

Drink - ______________________

Carbohydrates	**Protein**	**Fat**
Total crab grams -	Total protein grams -	Total fat grams -
Total fiber grams -	Total protein calories -	Total fat calories
Total sugar grams -		Total saturated
Total complex grams -		Total unsaturated -
Total carb calories -		

Total calories of meal - **cal**
Total ounces of water with meal - **ounces**
Total sodium of meal - **mgs**

Total ounces of water with meals - **ounces**
Total ounces of water during workout - **ounces**
Total ounces of water outside meals - **ounces**
Total ounces of water today - **ounces**
Total sodium today - **mgs**

Round 9 - Day 2

Do you ever wake up and wonder what day it is? I do it all the time and I think it's because I sleep so well. Good morning! Are you ready for some core and cardio today? I hope so, because ready or not, here it comes!

Which Way You Headed?

Write your three goals about things other than fitness, and below each one, write one obstacle you have overcome for each goal.

Goal 1 - ____

One obstacle I have overcome in reaching this goal is…

____

Goal 2 - ____

One obstacle I have overcome in reaching this goal is…

____

Goal 3 - ____

One obstacle I have overcome in reaching this goal is…

____

Seeing I to Eye

Here's a good one for you: Think of one of your all time favorite movies and once you got it, visualize yourself as a main character in that movie. Go ahead and have some fun with this one but you can't use *Braveheart*; that's mine. Okay; I'll share.

Upper Management

Remember that list you wrote of things you need to get done? You can also write daily list of things you need to do for that particular day. If I didn't do this, I would be in big trouble. You can use your phone, computer, or a notepad, and at the beginning of your day or the night before, just make a list of those things you need to do for that particular day. It sure makes things easier when you do it.

Your Workout – See your workout log for today's workout.

Cleaning Your Plate

Is it really such a big deal if you skip one of your meals?

Remember when we talked about eating 4-5 smaller meals a day? The reason you should do this is to keep your metabolism working at an optimum level by giving your body the right amount of nutrition at the right times. When your body goes without nutrition for an extended amount of time, it will slow everything down and conserve energy to make sure it has enough for your basic functions; this is what's called lowering your metabolism which nobody wants. This is exactly what happens if you skip a meal or if you only eat 1-2 meals a day.

So, my answer is…Yes, it's a big deal if you skip a meal. How about that for a rhyme?

You Ate What???

Are you eating 4-5 times a day? If you're not, make that move!

Food Journal

Time of meal 1 - _________

Food eaten- ____

Drink - ________________________

Carbohydrates		**Protein**		**Fat**	
Total crab grams -		Total protein grams -		Total fat grams -	
Total fiber grams -		Total protein calories -		Total fat calories	
Total sugar grams -				Total saturated	
Total complex grams -				Total unsaturated -	
Total carb calories -					
Percentage of meal -	%	Percentage of meal -	%	Percentage of meal -	%

Total calories of meal - **cal**
Total ounces of water with meal - **ounces**
Total sodium of meal - **mgs**

Time of meal 2 - _________

Food eaten- ____

Drink - ________________________

Carbohydrates		**Protein**		**Fat**	
Total crab grams -		Total protein grams -		Total fat grams -	
Total fiber grams -		Total protein calories -		Total fat calories	
Total sugar grams -				Total saturated	
Total complex grams -				Total unsaturated -	
Total carb calories -					
Percentage of meal -	%	Percentage of meal -	%	Percentage of meal -	%

Total calories of meal - **cal**
Total ounces of water with meal - **ounces**
Total sodium of meal - **mgs**

Time of meal 3 (Lunch) - _________

Food eaten- ____

Drink - ________________________

Carbohydrates	**Protein**	**Fat**
Total crab grams -	Total protein grams -	Total fat grams -
Total fiber grams -	Total protein calories -	Total fat calories
Total sugar grams -		Total saturated
Total complex grams -		Total unsaturated -
Total carb calories -		

Total calories of meal - **cal**
Total ounces of water with meal - **ounces**
Total sodium of meal - **mgs**

Time of meal 4 - _________

Food eaten- ____

Drink - ________________________

Carbohydrates	**Protein**	**Fat**
Total crab grams -	Total protein grams -	Total fat grams -
Total fiber grams -	Total protein calories -	Total fat calories
Total sugar grams -		Total saturated
Total complex grams -		Total unsaturated -
Total carb calories -		

Total calories of meal - **cal**
Total ounces of water with meal - **ounces**
Total sodium of meal - **mgs**

Time of meal 5 - ________

Food eaten- ____

Drink - ________________________

Carbohydrates	**Protein**	**Fat**
Total crab grams -	Total protein grams -	Total fat grams -
Total fiber grams -	Total protein calories -	Total fat calories
Total sugar grams -		Total saturated
Total complex grams -		Total unsaturated -
Total carb calories -		

Total calories of meal - **cal**
Total ounces of water with meal - **ounces**
Total sodium of meal - **mgs**

Total ounces of water with meals - **ounces**
Total ounces of water during workout - **ounces**
Total ounces of water outside meals - **ounces**
Total ounces of water today - **ounces**
Total sodium today - **mgs**

And The Heart Says…

At some point in the middle of your day, take a heart rate and record it here.

Afternoon HR-________ Time taken - _______

You've definitely stepped it up with Round 9. I'm talking about everything and not just your workouts. Your body and mind are getting stronger, and your confidence is stepping up to the plate as well. Keep it up!

Round 9 – Day 3

Before you get going today, I want you do to one thing: Take a minute and write down how you're energy has been effected with 12 Rounds up to this point.

Since I started 12 Rounds, my energy has…

____

That One Thing

On Day 1 of this round you wrote down one thing you've always wanted to do but are too shy or uncomfortable to do it. Today, write it again here along with one thing you can do to edge closer to actually doing it.

One thing I've always wanted to do but haven't drummed up the courage to actually do is…

____

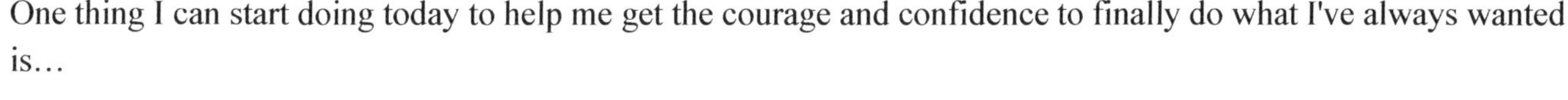

One thing I can start doing today to help me get the courage and confidence to finally do what I've always wanted is…

____

Seeing I to Eye

We all have those things in the back of our minds we worry about on a daily basis. Pick one of those things and spend 5-6 minutes today visualizing it turning out in a good way for you. This is very powerful so take your time, stay positive, and see it turning out great.

Your Workout – See your workout log for today's workout.

And the Heart Says…

While you're at work today and sitting at your desk, take a heart rate and write it down here. Make sure you've been sitting for at least 5 minutes before you take it. Also, take a look back at your first few rounds and see if there is a difference in your heart rates.

Resting HR - ______ Time Taken - ________

Cleaning Your Plate

How do I know for sure that the body weight I am losing is truly fat and not lean muscle mass?

This is a big one! The only way to truly know whether your losing fat, muscle, or both during your weight loss is to do the following:

- Get your body fat tested and know your body weight before you start your weight loss program
- Make sure the person taking your body fat has a lot of experience in doing this and they take it three times to ensure accuracy.
- Retest every two weeks.

If your body weight goes down, but your body fat % stays the same or even goes up, this means you are definitely losing lean muscle mass. If your body weight stays the same but your body fat % goes down, you've definitely lost body fat. And lastly, if your body weight goes down and your body fat % goes down as well, you're probably losing body fat and keeping your lean muscle mass.

This is the only way to truly know what kind of weight you're actually losing.

You Ate What???

For the last week or so, you've been taking percentages of the types of food you are eating for two meals a day. Let's add the rest of your meals to this and see how you're doing across the entire day. I also asked you to start shooting for a 40% carbs/30% protein/30% fat ratio for two of your meals. In addition, if you are trying to lose some body fat, start shooting for a 30% carbs/40% protein/30% fat ratio. To do this, just carve out a few more carbs from your later meals, replace those calories with protein, and keep your fats the same.

Food Journal

Time of meal 1 - _________

Food eaten- ____

Drink - ________________________

Carbohydrates		**Protein**		**Fat**	
Total crab grams -		Total protein grams -		Total fat grams -	
Total fiber grams -		Total protein calories -		Total fat calories	
Total sugar grams -				Total saturated	
Total complex grams -				Total unsaturated -	
Total carb calories -					
Percentage of meal -	%	Percentage of meal -	%	Percentage of meal -	%

Total calories of meal - **cal**
Total ounces of water with meal - **ounces**
Total sodium of meal - **mgs**

Time of meal 2 - _________

Food eaten- ____

Drink - ________________________

Carbohydrates		**Protein**		**Fat**	
Total crab grams -		Total protein grams -		Total fat grams -	
Total fiber grams -		Total protein calories -		Total fat calories	
Total sugar grams -				Total saturated	
Total complex grams -				Total unsaturated -	
Total carb calories -					
Percentage of meal -	%	Percentage of meal -	%	Percentage of meal -	%

Total calories of meal - **cal**
Total ounces of water with meal - **ounces**
Total sodium of meal - **mgs**

Time of meal 3 (Lunch) - _________

Food eaten- ____

Drink - ________________________

Carbohydrates		**Protein**		**Fat**	
Total crab grams -		Total protein grams -		Total fat grams -	
Total fiber grams -		Total protein calories -		Total fat calories	
Total sugar grams -				Total saturated	
Total complex grams -				Total unsaturated -	
Total carb calories -					
Percentage of meal -	%	Percentage of meal -	%	Percentage of meal -	%

Total calories of meal - **cal**
Total ounces of water with meal - **ounces**
Total sodium of meal - **mgs**

Time of meal 4 - _________

Food eaten- ____

Drink - ________________________

Carbohydrates		**Protein**		**Fat**	
Total crab grams -		Total protein grams -		Total fat grams -	
Total fiber grams -		Total protein calories -		Total fat calories	
Total sugar grams -				Total saturated	
Total complex grams -				Total unsaturated -	
Total carb calories -					
Percentage of meal -	%	Percentage of meal -	%	Percentage of meal -	%

Total calories of meal - **cal**
Total ounces of water with meal - **ounces**
Total sodium of meal - **mgs**

Time of meal 5 - _________

Food eaten- ____

Drink - ________________________

Carbohydrates		**Protein**		**Fat**	
Total crab grams -		Total protein grams -		Total fat grams -	
Total fiber grams -		Total protein calories -		Total fat calories	
Total sugar grams -				Total saturated	
Total complex grams -				Total unsaturated -	
Total carb calories -					
Percentage of meal -	%	Percentage of meal -	%	Percentage of meal -	%

Total calories of meal - **cal**
Total ounces of water with meal - **ounces**
Total sodium of meal - **mgs**

Total ounces of water with meals - **ounces**
Total ounces of water during workout - **ounces**
Total ounces of water outside meals - **ounces**
Total ounces of water today - **ounces**
Total sodium today - **mgs**

I know I have said this a few times before but your food journal is the most significant tool you have to get and maintain control of your body weight, your energy, and your overall health. That's why it takes recording all variables so you can see exactly where things may be off in your eating. Plus, you won't have to wonder why any more, right? Keep it up Champ, and I'll see you tomorrow.

Round 9 - Day 4

I know I call this your day off from exercise but other than giving your body a break, it allows you to exercise your mind in different ways. Round 9 is about building your confidence to do things you used to think you couldn't do, and I think you're doing awesome. Let's keep moving toward a stronger you and own this Day 4!

"You can spend a lot of your life thinking you can do something, or you can spend an eternity being proud and smiling because you actually did it." Bobby Whisnand

It Happened Just Like This!

One of the proudest moments in my life was from what someone else achieved. I had a client who was considerably overweight (about 120 pounds to be exact). She hired me to train her in her home and she made clear to me when we started that she hated going to the gym because she felt so out of place, embarrassed, and intimidated. This lady loved working out and she was damn good at it too, so one day I sat her down and said, "I think we need to set another goal right now. I'm going to teach you to jump rope and after you get it down, you and I are going to walk into a gym, start working out, and watch everyone's face when you break out that rope and jump it like a champ." She gave me a really weird look and after a few seconds she said, "I don't know how that's going to be possible because I don't think there's any way I could ever jump rope, but if you think I can, I'm in."

She started by doing one jump rope at a time and could only do about 4-5 of them for her first week, but that soon changed. Three months later we walked into a gym and she jumped rope like she weighed 110. I cannot tell you the looks of amazement going on from everywhere in that gym and at that moment, I was one proud trainer. We worked out for an hour, walked out, and she said in tears, "My life just changed before my very eyes. I just did three things I thought I'd never be able to do; worked out in a gym full of people, jumped rope, and felt like I was on top of the world.

Don't ever sell yourself short. Reach way down deep where your soul lives, hold on tight, and go get what you want out of life. And never let anyone talk you out of it.

Which Way You Headed?

Write your three goals about your fitness and below each one, write one obstacle you have overcome for each goal.

Goal 1 - ____

One obstacle I have overcome in reaching this goal is…

____

Goal 2 - ____

One obstacle I have overcome in reaching this goal is…

____

Goal 3 - ____

One obstacle I have overcome in reaching this goal is…

____

Seeing I to Eye

Let's get back to basics for this one day. I want you to really put your mind into this one. Get in that quiet place and visualize yourself the way you want to look physically. While you're at it, visualize yourself being very energetic, smiling, and even throw in one of your favorite upbeat songs. ACDC works great for me.

Upper Management

Make sure you are planning ahead for work projects, family activities, kids programs, and of course your workouts. When you fill out your schedule, give yourself plenty of transition time between appointments just in case something goes awry. Don't forget to have an alternate plan ready too; you know how things can happen.

No Workout Today!

And the Heart Says…

Take at least one heart rate today whenever you want. Just make sure you write down when and under what circumstances you took it.

Today I took my heart rate when I was… _____________________________________

Day 4 HR - ______ Time taken - ________

Cleaning Your Plate

If I'm having a tough time losing weight and managing my food, should I join one of those national weight loss programs?

I'm all for joining a weight loss program for several reasons: They provide instant accountability, they help you track and manage your eating, and they have prepared meals which makes it easier for you to stay on your eating plan. But, there are things you should watch out for, and I have listed them here:

- Stay away from any program that says, "No exercise needed".
- Do your research online and look for comments and success stories about the program you are considering.
- Ask to see the qualifications of their nutritionist or food counselors and make sure they are truly capable of helping you in the right ways.
- Make sure you know all of the expenses of joining the program including the cost of the meals.

You Ate What???

How's it going? Are you getting close to the 40/30/30 ratio or have you made your move to the 30/40/30 ratio? Either way, keep up the good work!

Food Journal

Time of meal 1 - _________

Food eaten- ____

Drink - ________________________

Carbohydrates		**Protein**		**Fat**	
Total crab grams -		Total protein grams -		Total fat grams -	
Total fiber grams -		Total protein calories -		Total fat calories	
Total sugar grams -				Total saturated	
Total complex grams -				Total unsaturated -	
Total carb calories -					
Percentage of meal -	%	Percentage of meal -	%	Percentage of meal -	%

Total calories of meal - **cal**
Total ounces of water with meal - **ounces**
Total sodium of meal - **mgs**

Time of meal 2 - _________

Food eaten- ____

Drink - ________________________

Carbohydrates		**Protein**		**Fat**	
Total crab grams -		Total protein grams -		Total fat grams -	
Total fiber grams -		Total protein calories -		Total fat calories	
Total sugar grams -				Total saturated	
Total complex grams -				Total unsaturated -	
Total carb calories -					
Percentage of meal -	%	Percentage of meal -	%	Percentage of meal -	%

Total calories of meal - **cal**
Total ounces of water with meal - **ounces**
Total sodium of meal - **mgs**

Time of meal 3 (Lunch) - _________

Food eaten- ____

Drink - ________________________

Carbohydrates		**Protein**		**Fat**	
Total crab grams -		Total protein grams -		Total fat grams -	
Total fiber grams -		Total protein calories -		Total fat calories	
Total sugar grams -				Total saturated	
Total complex grams -				Total unsaturated -	
Total carb calories -					
Percentage of meal -	%	Percentage of meal -	%	Percentage of meal -	%

Total calories of meal - **cal**
Total ounces of water with meal - **ounces**
Total sodium of meal - **mgs**

Time of meal 4 - ________

Food eaten- ____

Drink - ________________________

Carbohydrates		**Protein**		**Fat**	
Total crab grams -		Total protein grams -		Total fat grams -	
Total fiber grams -		Total protein calories -		Total fat calories	
Total sugar grams -				Total saturated	
Total complex grams -				Total unsaturated -	
Total carb calories -					
Percentage of meal -	%	Percentage of meal -	%	Percentage of meal -	%

Total calories of meal - **cal**
Total ounces of water with meal - **ounces**
Total sodium of meal - **mgs**

Time of meal 5 - ________

Food eaten- ____

Drink - ________________________

Carbohydrates		**Protein**		**Fat**	
Total crab grams -		Total protein grams -		Total fat grams -	
Total fiber grams -		Total protein calories -		Total fat calories	
Total sugar grams -				Total saturated	
Total complex grams -				Total unsaturated -	
Total carb calories -					
Percentage of meal -	%	Percentage of meal -	%	Percentage of meal -	%

Total calories of meal - **cal**
Total ounces of water with meal - **ounces**
Total sodium of meal - **mgs**

Total ounces of water with meals - **ounces**
Total ounces of water during workout - **ounces**
Total ounces of water outside meals - **ounces**
Total ounces of water today - **ounces**
Total sodium today - **mgs**

Great job today! Don't forget to drink plenty of water, watch that sodium intake, and clear that head so you can get some great sleep. I'll see you tomorrow for back and biceps.

Round 9 - Day 5

Get on up and let's go. Your back and biceps know what day it is; don't let them down. Don't forget your water first thing when you get up and definitely don't skip that breakfast. I'll see you in the gym!

That One Thing

On Day 1, you wrote down one thing you want to do, but you're not confident enough to do it. On Day 3 you wrote down one thing you could do to help you get closer to actually doing it. Today, write both of these down again and in addition, write one more thing you can do to help you get the courage to do this elusive thing.

One thing I've always wanted to do but haven't drummed up the courage to actually do is…

____

One thing I can start doing today to help me get the courage and confidence to finally do what I really want to is…

____

Another thing I can do to help me get the courage and confidence to do this thing is…

____

Seeing I to Eye

Think of a competition you'd like to win and take 5-6 minutes today seeing yourself take the prize. It could be something physical, a sales contest at work, fishing tournament (yep, that's mine), dance contest, political office, or anything else you want to win. See it, feel it, hear it, and make it yours!

Your Workout – See your workout log for today's workout.

And the Heart Says…

Sometime after dinner and when you have been relaxing for about an hour, take and record a heart rate. Start looking back at your earlier rounds and see what's changed with your heart rates.

Evening resting HR ______ Time taken ______

Cleaning Your Plate

Is it okay to skip lunch and workout instead?

Absolutely not! It's definitely okay to work out over your lunch time but make sure you eat your lunch as soon as you get back to work. This is where making your meals ahead of time really pays off. You can go workout during your lunch hour, come back to work, and simply heat up your lunch and eat it right at your desk if you have to. Whatever you do: Don't Skip Meals!

You Ate What???

I know we are journaling a lot, but I want to remind you of a few things you need to keep your eyes on.

- Read those ingredients and know what's in your food and how it was made.

- Stay away from processed foods and only eat whole natural foods.
- Make half your plate vegetables and also eat 4-5 servings of fruit a day.
- Watch out for sodium; it can add up fast!
- Eat plenty of good fats (30% of your diet).
- If you're trying to lose weight, get rid of those complex starchy carbs later in your day.

Food Journal

Time of meal 1 - _________

Food eaten- ____

Drink - ________________________

Carbohydrates	**Protein**	**Fat**
Total crab grams -	Total protein grams -	Total fat grams -
Total fiber grams -	Total protein calories -	Total fat calories
Total sugar grams -		Total saturated
Total complex grams -		Total unsaturated -
Total carb calories -		
Percentage of meal - %	Percentage of meal - %	Percentage of meal - %

Total calories of meal - cal
Total ounces of water with meal - ounces
Total sodium of meal - mgs

Time of meal 2 - _________

Food eaten- ____

Drink - ________________________

Carbohydrates	**Protein**	**Fat**
Total crab grams -	Total protein grams -	Total fat grams -
Total fiber grams -	Total protein calories -	Total fat calories
Total sugar grams -		Total saturated
Total complex grams -		Total unsaturated -
Total carb calories -		
Percentage of meal - %	Percentage of meal - %	Percentage of meal - %

Total calories of meal - cal
Total ounces of water with meal - ounces
Total sodium of meal - mgs

Time of meal 3 (Lunch) - _________

Food eaten- ____

Drink - ________________________

Carbohydrates		**Protein**		**Fat**	
Total crab grams -		Total protein grams -		Total fat grams -	
Total fiber grams -		Total protein calories -		Total fat calories	
Total sugar grams -				Total saturated	
Total complex grams -				Total unsaturated -	
Total carb calories -					
Percentage of meal -	%	Percentage of meal -	%	Percentage of meal -	%

Total calories of meal - cal
Total ounces of water with meal - ounces
Total sodium of meal - mgs

Time of meal 4 - _________

Food eaten- ____

Drink - ________________________

Carbohydrates		**Protein**		**Fat**	
Total crab grams -		Total protein grams -		Total fat grams -	
Total fiber grams -		Total protein calories -		Total fat calories	
Total sugar grams -				Total saturated	
Total complex grams -				Total unsaturated -	
Total carb calories -					
Percentage of meal -	%	Percentage of meal -	%	Percentage of meal -	%

Total calories of meal - cal
Total ounces of water with meal - ounces
Total sodium of meal - mgs

Time of meal 5 - _________

Food eaten- ____

Drink - ________________________

Carbohydrates		**Protein**		**Fat**	
Total crab grams -		Total protein grams -		Total fat grams -	
Total fiber grams -		Total protein calories -		Total fat calories	
Total sugar grams -				Total saturated	
Total complex grams -				Total unsaturated -	
Total carb calories -					
Percentage of meal -	%	Percentage of meal -	%	Percentage of meal -	%

Total calories of meal - cal
Total ounces of water with meal - ounces
Total sodium of meal - mgs

Total ounces of water with meals - ounces
Total ounces of water during workout - ounces
Total ounces of water outside meals - ounces
Total ounces of water today - ounces
Total sodium today - mgs

How about it? Are you ready to finish your day and get to Day 6? Go take it easy, watch something good on T.V., and think about a few of your goals before you go to bed and what you need to do to reach them. Make sure you also take a look at your workout for tomorrow; it's one you're not soon to forget.

Round 9 - Day 6

Day 6; core, cardio, and one step closer to reaching your goals. I'm not going to hold you back; go get after it!

Which Way You Headed?

Write your three goals about your career and below each one, write one obstacle you have overcome for each goal.

Goal 1 - ____

One obstacle I have overcome in reaching this goal is…

____

Goal 2 - ____

One obstacle I have overcome in reaching this goal is…

____

Goal 3 - ____

One obstacle I have overcome in reaching this goal is…

____

Upper Management

If you have an unsettled situation with a friend, co-worker, or family member, take the initiative and talk with that person and work towards a resolution. If they are unwilling to talk, walk away and try again at a different time, but don't give up on them. These are the very things that can wreck your whole day, week, or month so fix things now so nobody has to fix you later.

Seeing I to Eye

On Days 1, 3, and 5, you wrote down one thing you want to do, but you don't have the confidence and courage to do it. Take 5-6 minutes today and visualize doing it and doing it well. I know you can do it, but for you to really be able to do it, you're going to have to see yourself do it first. While you're at it, visualize those two things you wrote down that can help you get it done. You are far more capable than you know.

Your Workout – See your workout log for today's workout.

And the Heart Says…

At some point this evening when you are relaxed, take another heart rate and record it here.

Post workout evening HR ______ Time taken __________

Cleaning Your Plate

Are diet sodas bad to drink?

Drinking a reasonable amount of diet soda a day, such as a can or two, isn't likely to hurt you. The artificial sweeteners and other chemicals currently used in diet soda are safe for most people, and there's no credible evidence that these ingredients cause cancer. But diet soda isn't a health drink or a silver bullet for weight loss. Although switching from regular soda to diet soda may save you calories in the short term, it's not yet clear if it's effective for preventing obesity and related health problems such as metabolic syndrome. I think you should stick as close to drinking water as you can and avoid anything artificial. Like I stated earlier, a little here and there is unlikely to hurt you, but anything in excess can cause health issues in one way or another.

You Ate What???

Are you starting to make changes with your individual meals like changing the percentages of carbs, proteins, and fats? Like I said earlier, if you're trying to lose weight, start reducing your carbohydrate calories and if your fat percentages are over 30%, start reducing these as well. Your total calories might be right on, but the calories distribution may be way off.

Food Journal

Time of meal 1 - _________

Food eaten- ____

Drink - ________________________

Carbohydrates		**Protein**		**Fat**	
Total crab grams -		Total protein grams -		Total fat grams -	
Total fiber grams -		Total protein calories -		Total fat calories	
Total sugar grams -				Total saturated	
Total complex grams -				Total unsaturated -	
Total carb calories -					
Percentage of meal -	%	Percentage of meal -	%	Percentage of meal -	%

Total calories of meal - **cal**
Total ounces of water with meal - **ounces**
Total sodium of meal - **mgs**

Time of meal 2 - _________

Food eaten- ____

Drink - ________________________

Carbohydrates	**Protein**	**Fat**
Total crab grams -	Total protein grams -	Total fat grams -
Total fiber grams -	Total protein calories -	Total fat calories
Total sugar grams -		Total saturated
Total complex grams -		Total unsaturated -
Total carb calories -		
Percentage of meal - %	Percentage of meal - %	Percentage of meal -

Total calories of meal - cal
Total ounces of water with meal - ounces
Total sodium of meal - mgs

Time of meal 3 (Lunch) - _________

Food eaten- ____

Drink - ________________________

Carbohydrates	**Protein**	**Fat**
Total crab grams -	Total protein grams -	Total fat grams -
Total fiber grams -	Total protein calories -	Total fat calories
Total sugar grams -		Total saturated
Total complex grams -		Total unsaturated -
Total carb calories -		
Percentage of meal - %	Percentage of meal - %	Percentage of meal - %

Total calories of meal - cal
Total ounces of water with meal - ounces
Total sodium of meal - mgs

Time of meal 4 - _________

Food eaten- ____

Drink - ________________________

Carbohydrates	**Protein**	**Fat**
Total crab grams -	Total protein grams -	Total fat grams -
Total fiber grams -	Total protein calories -	Total fat calories
Total sugar grams -		Total saturated
Total complex grams -		Total unsaturated -
Total carb calories -		
Percentage of meal - %	Percentage of meal - %	Percentage of meal - %

Total calories of meal - cal
Total ounces of water with meal - ounces
Total sodium of meal - mgs

Time of meal 5 - _________

Food eaten- ____

Drink - ________________________

Carbohydrates	**Protein**	**Fat**
Total crab grams -	Total protein grams -	Total fat grams -
Total fiber grams -	Total protein calories -	Total fat calories
Total sugar grams -		Total saturated
Total complex grams -		Total unsaturated -
Total carb calories -		
Percentage of meal - %	Percentage of meal - %	Percentage of meal - %

Total calories of meal - cal
Total ounces of water with meal - ounces
Total sodium of meal - mgs

Total ounces of water with meals - ounces
Total ounces of water during workout - ounces
Total ounces of water outside meals - ounces
Total ounces of water today - ounces
Total sodium today - mgs

Can you believe you've almost completed Round 9? That's just crazy! After tomorrow, you'll be entering the home stretch and I promise to make it the best three rounds yet. Go ahead; enjoy your progress and I'll see you tomorrow for Day 7.

Round 9- Day 7

I hope you are proud of yourself. 12 Rounds isn't just another new workout fad that you do for a while and then watch as it fades away. It's 12 weeks of making real productive changes in your health, your state of mind, your well being, and your confidence that will stick with you for the rest of your life. Enjoy yourself today and get ready for the final three rounds.

I took this heart rate when I was…____

Day 7 HR ______ Time taken _______

Food Journal

Time of meal 1 - _________

Food eaten- ____

Drink - _________________________

Carbohydrates	**Protein**	**Fat**
Total crab grams -	Total protein grams -	Total fat grams -
Total fiber grams -	Total protein calories -	Total fat calories
Total sugar grams -		Total saturated
Total complex grams -		Total unsaturated -
Total carb calories -		
Percentage of meal - %	Percentage of meal - %	Percentage of meal - %

Total calories of meal - cal
Total ounces of water with meal - ounces
Total sodium of meal - mgs

Time of meal 2 - ________

Food eaten- ____

Drink - ________________________

Carbohydrates		**Protein**		**Fat**	
Total crab grams -		Total protein grams -		Total fat grams -	
Total fiber grams -		Total protein calories -		Total fat calories	
Total sugar grams -				Total saturated	
Total complex grams -				Total unsaturated -	
Total carb calories -					
Percentage of meal -	%	Percentage of meal -	%	Percentage of meal -	%
Total calories of meal -		**cal**			
Total ounces of water with meal -		**ounces**			
Total sodium of meal -		**mgs**			

Time of meal 3 (Lunch) - ________

Food eaten- ____

Drink - ________________________

Carbohydrates		**Protein**		**Fat**	
Total crab grams -		Total protein grams -		Total fat grams -	
Total fiber grams -		Total protein calories -		Total fat calories	
Total sugar grams -				Total saturated	
Total complex grams -				Total unsaturated -	
Total carb calories -					
Percentage of meal -	%	Percentage of meal -	%	Percentage of meal -	%
Total calories of meal -		**cal**			
Total ounces of water with meal -		**ounces**			
Total sodium of meal -		**mgs**			

Time of meal 4 - ________

Food eaten- ____

Drink - ________________________

Carbohydrates		**Protein**		**Fat**	
Total crab grams -		Total protein grams -		Total fat grams -	
Total fiber grams -		Total protein calories -		Total fat calories	
Total sugar grams -				Total saturated	
Total complex grams -				Total unsaturated -	
Total carb calories -					
Percentage of meal -	%	Percentage of meal -	%	Percentage of meal -	%
Total calories of meal -		**cal**			
Total ounces of water with meal -		**ounces**			
Total sodium of meal -		**mgs**			

Time of meal 5 - _________

Food eaten- ____

Drink - ________________________

Carbohydrates		**Protein**		**Fat**	
Total crab grams -		Total protein grams -		Total fat grams -	
Total fiber grams -		Total protein calories -		Total fat calories	
Total sugar grams -				Total saturated	
Total complex grams -				Total unsaturated -	
Total carb calories -					
Percentage of meal -	%	Percentage of meal -	%	Percentage of meal -	%

Total calories of meal - **cal**
Total ounces of water with meal - **ounces**
Total sodium of meal - **mgs**

Total ounces of water with meals - **ounces**
Total ounces of water during workout - **ounces**
Total ounces of water outside meals - **ounces**
Total ounces of water today - **ounces**
Total sodium today - **mgs**

Round 10 – Giving Back

Day 1

Hey Champ! What do you say we take this thing to a whole new level? I'm not talking about exercise this time; I'm talking about making someone else's heart swell by giving back. This is what takes up more room in my heart than anything else and I hope you feel the same. Let's make Round 10 the best yet!

"A heart of gold is not made from money; it's made from giving pieces of your own heart to as many people as you can, never worrying about how much you'll have left to give, and never asking for anything in return."
Bobby Whisnand

It Happened Just Like This!

I've given a lot of presentations over the years and I've made some great memories, but there was one that affected me in a way I'll never forget. I was speaking to a very small church in south Dallas on Valentine's weekend. This little church would only hold about 100 people and about 200 showed up for my presentation. Most of my audience was ladies dressed in their Sunday finest with big colorful hats, long fancy gloves, and beautiful dresses. As they introduced me, they made me an honorary member of their church and presented me with a very nice framed and glassed certificate. After my presentation, every single one of them lined up, shook my hand or hugged me, introduced themselves, told me how much they appreciated me, took pictures with me, and asked me to stay and eat with them. And to top that off, they gave me a very nice pen set and again thanked me for my time.

That was the most appreciative audience I've ever presented to, and even though they didn't have much in the way of money, they made sure I knew how much they appreciated me. Oh, and the food I got to eat...let's just say I gained a few pounds before I left that church and didn't eat for the next several hours.

That One Thing

Over the next two days, find one place where you can volunteer to help those less fortunate and make a plan to get involved. There are countless places that would love to have your help like homeless shelters, homes for abused women and children, long term care facilities, schools, and many others. Find that place and write it down here.

The place where I am going to volunteer and give my time is...

____

Seeing I to Eye

Think about someone you know who is going though something very trying. Once you have them in your head, visualize how you would respond if it was you in their shoes. This might start out a little sad for you, but you have the ability to make it end with a positive outcome.

Your Workout – See your workout log for today's workout.

And the Heart Says...

After you take this heart rate, take a look back at your heart rates during the first two rounds and see what the difference is.

Pre Sleep HR - ______ Time taken ________

Cleaning Your Plate

What exactly does it mean to a vegetarian and Vegan ,and is there a difference?

Vegetarianism has been practiced for many centuries. Some are vegetarian for religious reasons, others for ethical reasons, and others simply believe that it is a healthier way to live. Some people believe that the words "vegetarian" and "vegan" mean the same thing, but they do not. Vegetarian is a broader term that encompasses several different diets, while vegans eat a specific type of diet and often try to avoid any animal products in their lives.

Vegans do not eat any type of animal flesh, nor do they consume animal products such as eggs and milk. Most vegans do not even eat honey, and some do not eat yeast products. Lifestyle characteristics include not wearing any type of animal product, including silk or wool, and not using lotions or other products that have ingredients that originate from animals.

These requirements are set forth by vegan societies. Individual vegans may or may not follow them to the letter, but the principle is to avoid consuming or using anything that could harm any type of animal. Those who adhere to a strict vegan diet but are not concerned with non-food uses of animal products are called dietary vegans.

You Ate What???

No changes today, but really start taking a close look at those percentages of carbs, proteins, and fats you're eating. Again, a 40/30/30 ratio is good, but if you are trying to shed some pounds and keep that lean muscle at the same time, try a 30/40/30 ratio.

Food Journal

Time of meal 1 - _________

Food eaten- ____

Drink - ________________________

Carbohydrates	**Protein**	**Fat**
Total crab grams -	Total protein grams -	Total fat grams -
Total fiber grams -	Total protein calories -	Total fat calories
Total sugar grams -		Total saturated
Total complex grams -		Total unsaturated -
Total carb calories -		
Percentage of meal - %	Percentage of meal - %	Percentage of meal - %

Total calories of meal - cal
Total ounces of water with meal - ounces
Total sodium of meal - mgs

Time of meal 2 - _________

Food eaten- ____

Drink - ________________________

Carbohydrates		**Protein**		**Fat**	
Total crab grams -		Total protein grams -		Total fat grams -	
Total fiber grams -		Total protein calories -		Total fat calories	
Total sugar grams -				Total saturated	
Total complex grams -				Total unsaturated -	
Total carb calories -					
Percentage of meal -	%	Percentage of meal -	%	Percentage of meal -	%

Total calories of meal - **cal**
Total ounces of water with meal - **ounces**
Total sodium of meal - **mgs**

Time of meal 3 (Lunch) - _________

Food eaten- ____

Drink - ________________________

Carbohydrates		**Protein**		**Fat**	
Total crab grams -		Total protein grams -		Total fat grams -	
Total fiber grams -		Total protein calories -		Total fat calories	
Total sugar grams -				Total saturated	
Total complex grams -				Total unsaturated -	
Total carb calories -					
Percentage of meal -	%	Percentage of meal -	%	Percentage of meal -	%

Total calories of meal - **cal**
Total ounces of water with meal - **ounces**
Total sodium of meal - **mgs**

Time of meal 4 - _________

Food eaten- ____

Drink - ________________________

Carbohydrates		**Protein**		**Fat**	
Total crab grams -		Total protein grams -		Total fat grams -	
Total fiber grams -		Total protein calories -		Total fat calories	
Total sugar grams -				Total saturated	
Total complex grams -				Total unsaturated -	
Total carb calories -					
Percentage of meal -	%	Percentage of meal -	%	Percentage of meal -	%

Total calories of meal - **cal**
Total ounces of water with meal - **ounces**
Total sodium of meal - **mgs**

Time of meal 5 - _________

Food eaten- ____

Drink - ________________________

Carbohydrates		**Protein**		**Fat**	
Total crab grams -		Total protein grams -		Total fat grams -	
Total fiber grams -		Total protein calories -		Total fat calories	
Total sugar grams -				Total saturated	
Total complex grams -				Total unsaturated -	
Total carb calories -					
Percentage of meal -	%	Percentage of meal -	%	Percentage of meal -	%

Total calories of meal - cal
Total ounces of water with meal - ounces
Total sodium of meal - mgs

Total ounces of water with meals - ounces
Total ounces of water during workout - ounces
Total ounces of water outside meals - ounces
Total ounces of water today - ounces
Total sodium today - mgs

Good job today! I told you Round 10 would be different. There's not a better feeling in the world than helping someone have a better life so feel good about what you're doing this round. Okay, go rest up; you've got a tough core and cardio workout tomorrow. Don't forget about that water, and I'll see you in the morning!

Round 10 - Day 2

How are you feeling this morning? Do you have any soreness in your chest, shoulders, and triceps? If you do, make sure it's not lasting more than 72 hours and if it is lasting longer, reduce the amount of weight you are using. Let's go give your core a workout!

Which Way You Headed?

Think about someone you know who could use some help setting a few goals. Once you know who it is, see if you can get them to set one goal about something other than fitness. If they agree, get them to write it down and put it where they will see it every day.

Seeing I to Eye

I know public speaking may not be your thing, but take 5-6 minutes today and visualize standing in front of a group of people telling them something you have learned from 12 Rounds. This can be a lot of things like eating better, exercising with good form, setting goals, or managing their stress. Be sure to see your audience smiling about what you're telling them.

Upper Management

It's very easy in life to get to a point where you feel overwhelmed because things have stacked up on you. The best way to keep this from happening or to get this feeling to go away is to make lists. You've had one of those lists from early on in 12 Rounds, and I suggested you make daily list as well. How are you doing with getting those things done and out of your mind? If you still have things on that list, make it a point to get them done so you can start with a clean slate.

Your Workout – See your workout log for today's workout.

Cleaning Your Plate

What exactly is the Paleo diet?

The Paleo diet, also nicknamed the caveman diet, primal diet, Stone Age diet, and hunter-gatherer diet runs on the same foods our hunter-gather ancestors supposedly ate: fruits, vegetables, meats, seafood, and nuts. This way of eating also encourages you to stay away from dairy, grains, processed food, legumes, starches, and alcohol. There are many people who currently use this way of eating and have gotten good results but there are many experts that say it's not the way to eat.

In my opinion, I have always believed unprocessed complex carbohydrates that come from grains should be a part of everyone's diet, unless they have an allergy to them. The amount of complex carbs you eat need to be measured and controlled but you still need them in your diet. I like the fact that the Paleo diet discourages eating processed foods, and encourages good fats and proteins but I will always suggest complex carbs be a part of everyone's diet.

You Ate What???

How close are you getting to that 40/30/30 ratio? That means you're eating 40% carbs, 30% protein, and 30% fat of your total daily calories. Also, keep a close eye on those sweet foods like sodas, sweeteners, and baked goods that can add a ton of empty calories to your diet. Do you remember talking about empty calories?

Food Journal

Time of meal 1 - _________

Food eaten- ____

Drink - ________________________

Carbohydrates	**Protein**	**Fat**
Total crab grams -	Total protein grams -	Total fat grams -
Total fiber grams -	Total protein calories -	Total fat calories
Total sugar grams -		Total saturated
Total complex grams -		Total unsaturated -
Total carb calories -		
Percentage of meal - %	Percentage of meal - %	Percentage of meal - %

Total calories of meal - **cal**
Total ounces of water with meal - **ounces**
Total sodium of meal - **mgs**

Time of meal 2 - _________

Food eaten- ____

Drink - ________________________

Carbohydrates		**Protein**		**Fat**	
Total crab grams -		Total protein grams -		Total fat grams -	
Total fiber grams -		Total protein calories -		Total fat calories	
Total sugar grams -				Total saturated	
Total complex grams -				Total unsaturated -	
Total carb calories -					
Percentage of meal -	%	Percentage of meal -	%	Percentage of meal -	%

Total calories of meal - **cal**
Total ounces of water with meal - **ounces**
Total sodium of meal - **mgs**

Time of meal 3 (Lunch) - _________

Food eaten- ____

Drink - ________________________

Carbohydrates		**Protein**		**Fat**	
Total crab grams -		Total protein grams -		Total fat grams -	
Total fiber grams -		Total protein calories -		Total fat calories	
Total sugar grams -				Total saturated	
Total complex grams -				Total unsaturated -	
Total carb calories -					
Percentage of meal -	%	Percentage of meal -	%	Percentage of meal -	%

Total calories of meal - **cal**
Total ounces of water with meal - **ounces**
Total sodium of meal - **mgs**

Time of meal 4 - _________

Food eaten- ____

Drink - ________________________

Carbohydrates		**Protein**		**Fat**	
Total crab grams -		Total protein grams -		Total fat grams -	
Total fiber grams -		Total protein calories -		Total fat calories	
Total sugar grams -				Total saturated	
Total complex grams -				Total unsaturated -	
Total carb calories -					
Percentage of meal -	%	Percentage of meal -	%	Percentage of meal -	%

Total calories of meal - **cal**
Total ounces of water with meal - **ounces**
Total sodium of meal - **mgs**

Time of meal 5 - ________

Food eaten- ____

Drink - ________________________

Carbohydrates	**Protein**	**Fat**
Total crab grams -	Total protein grams -	Total fat grams -
Total fiber grams -	Total protein calories -	Total fat calories
Total sugar grams -		Total saturated
Total complex grams -		Total unsaturated -
Total carb calories -		
Percentage of meal - %	Percentage of meal - %	Percentage of meal - %

Total calories of meal - cal
Total ounces of water with meal - ounces
Total sodium of meal - mgs

Total ounces of water with meals - ounces
Total ounces of water during workout - ounces
Total ounces of water outside meals - ounces
Total ounces of water today - ounces
Total sodium today - mgs

And The Heart Says…

At some point in the middle of your day, take a heart rate and record it here. Start taking a look back through your earlier rounds and see what changes are happening with your heart rates.

Afternoon HR-_______ **Time taken -** _______

Remember, if you are trying to lose body fat, make sure you eat very little complex carbs later in your day, especially at dinner. Stick with lean protein and green vegetables for dinner and you will definitely shed that body fat while you sleep. Tomorrow's a big day so rest up; your legs are going to need it.

Round 10 – Day 3

I've got a great day planned for you but before we get going, I want you to answer a few questions for me.

- How many hours of sleep did you get last night? _______ hours
- How much water did you drink yesterday? _______ounces
- Did you think about something positive before you went to sleep last night? _______
- Has your energy increased since you started 12 Rounds? _______

That One Thing

Think of one person who needs help finishing something. It could be a friend, co-worker, or family member who needs a little help checking something off of their list. Once you know who it is, call them and tell them you want to help and make a plan to get it done together.

Seeing I to Eye

Think about some of the material things you have and how they make you feel to have them. Now visualize yourself without any of these things and see how this makes you feel. Can you still find a way to see yourself being happy? This is a tough one so take all the time you need, but as always, finish on a positive note.

Your Workout – See your workout log for today's workout.

And the Heart Says…

While you're at work today and sitting at your desk, take a heart rate and write it down here. Make sure you've been sitting for at least 5 minutes before you take it. Also, take a look back at your first few rounds and see if there is a difference in your heart rates.

Resting HR - ______ Time Taken - ________

Cleaning Your Plate

If I hit a plateau in my weight loss or weight gain, should I change something?

Regardless of whether you're trying to lose or gain weight, the first thing you want to do is make sure you're truly hitting a plateau. If you've gone two weeks without a change in weight, I would change just a few small things, journal these changes, and give it a week or so to see if things start to change for you. Try subtracting or adding calories to your overall eating plan, adding or reducing the amount of cardio activity you do, and take a long hard look at your food journal to see where you may be making a few mistakes.

The key is to only make a few small changes, journal what changes you've made, and watch closely for things to change.

You Ate What???

Take a close look at the total calories for each of your meals. A good idea is to have roughly the same amount of calories for breakfast and lunch, and fewer calories for your snack meals and dinner. Try to spread the calories out across the course of your day and don't eat too much at once.

Food Journal

Time of meal 1 - _________

Food eaten- ____

Drink - ________________________

Carbohydrates		**Protein**		**Fat**	
Total crab grams -		Total protein grams -		Total fat grams -	
Total fiber grams -		Total protein calories -		Total fat calories	
Total sugar grams -				Total saturated	
Total complex grams -				Total unsaturated -	
Total carb calories -					
Percentage of meal -	%	Percentage of meal -	%	Percentage of meal -	%

Total calories of meal - **cal**
Total ounces of water with meal - **ounces**
Total sodium of meal - **mgs**

Time of meal 2 - _________

Food eaten- ____

Drink - ________________________

Carbohydrates		**Protein**		**Fat**	
Total crab grams -		Total protein grams -		Total fat grams -	
Total fiber grams -		Total protein calories -		Total fat calories	
Total sugar grams -				Total saturated	
Total complex grams -				Total unsaturated -	
Total carb calories -					
Percentage of meal -	%	Percentage of meal -	%	Percentage of meal -	%

Total calories of meal - **cal**
Total ounces of water with meal - **ounces**
Total sodium of meal - **mgs**

Time of meal 3 (Lunch) - _________

Food eaten- ____

Drink - ________________________

Carbohydrates		**Protein**		**Fat**	
Total crab grams -		Total protein grams -		Total fat grams -	
Total fiber grams -		Total protein calories -		Total fat calories	
Total sugar grams -				Total saturated	
Total complex grams -				Total unsaturated -	
Total carb calories -					
Percentage of meal -	%	Percentage of meal -	%	Percentage of meal -	%

Total calories of meal - **cal**
Total ounces of water with meal - **ounces**
Total sodium of meal - **mgs**

Time of meal 4 - _________

Food eaten- ____

Drink - ________________________

Carbohydrates		**Protein**		**Fat**	
Total crab grams -		Total protein grams -		Total fat grams -	
Total fiber grams -		Total protein calories -		Total fat calories	
Total sugar grams -				Total saturated	
Total complex grams -				Total unsaturated -	
Total carb calories -					
Percentage of meal -	%	Percentage of meal -	%	Percentage of meal -	%

Total calories of meal - **cal**
Total ounces of water with meal - **ounces**
Total sodium of meal - **mgs**

Time of meal 5 - _________

Food eaten- ____

Drink - ________________________

Carbohydrates		**Protein**		**Fat**	
Total crab grams -		Total protein grams -		Total fat grams -	
Total fiber grams -		Total protein calories -		Total fat calories	
Total sugar grams -				Total saturated	
Total complex grams -				Total unsaturated -	
Total carb calories -					
Percentage of meal -	%	Percentage of meal -	%	Percentage of meal -	%

Total calories of meal - **cal**
Total ounces of water with meal - **ounces**
Total sodium of meal - **mgs**

Total ounces of water with meals - **ounces**
Total ounces of water during workout - **ounces**
Total ounces of water outside meals - **ounces**
Total ounces of water today - **ounces**
Total sodium today - **mgs**

Tonight before you go to bed, spend about 10 minutes looking through your food journal from the past few rounds and see where you're making great choices. While you're at it, make a few notes on where you can improve your eating. Other than that, think about something good before you fall to sleep and I'll see you tomorrow for Day 4.

Round 10 - Day 4

Here's another one of those days off for you. I guess it's not really a day off because you still have to train your brain a bit and journal your food, but the exercise stuff is put off for another day. Let's go make this day a good one!

"It's not the size, cost, or amount of a gift given; it's the size of the heart behind the gift that makes it priceless" Bobby Whisnand

It Happened Just Like This!

One of the biggest acts of kindness I've ever seen happened to me at my first book signing a few months back. My family, old high school friends, and many of my dad's friends came to hear my story and to get a copy of my very first book. My Dad asked me if I saw a particular friend of his, and I told him I did and that he bought a book. He then told me his friend was really having a hard time; his wife was in the middle of cancer treatment, he had just lost his job, his vehicle had broken down, and he had to get a ride to my book signing. The first thing that popped into my head was the fact that this man during a time of destitution put all of his hardships aside, found a way to come see me, and gave me $20 for one of my books; all when he had an overwhelming need for money. That man set aside his many problems and put my interest and my feelings in front of his.

He had left before I could catch him, so the very next weekend I drove back to my hometown, went to this man's house, gave him the twenty dollars back, and my dad and I both gave him a little extra to get by for a while. He and his wife tried very hard to not take the money, but I finally got my way. The gratitude I saw from both of their faces through their tears will be etched in my heart forever.

Which Way You Headed?

On Day 1, you were to help someone set a goal about something other than their fitness. Today, help that same person or find another person and help them write a goal about their fitness. This is a great opportunity to share your goals with them so they can see how you did it. You can also show them your progress and maybe motivate them to get on their way to improving their lives too.

Seeing I to Eye

Take some time today and think back to a point in your life when you put someone else's needs in front of yours. Spend some time visualizing this experience and if you want, think of a few times when you've done this. While you're visualizing these wonderful experiences, soak them up in your soul.

Upper Management

This round is about giving back and I've got a great way for you to do just that. Find a way to make a donation over the next several days. It could be donating clothes to the Salvation Army; it could be a monetary donation to a charity, donating blood, or simply donating your time to a needy cause for children or others in need.

No Workout Today!

And the Heart Says…

Take at least one heart rate today whenever you want. Just make sure you write down when and under what circumstances you took it.

Today I took my heart rate when I was... ____

Day 4 HR - ______ Time taken - ________

Cleaning Your Plate

What exactly is it that causes diabetes?

First of all I want to clarify the difference between Type 1 and Type 2 diabetes. In general, people with diabetes either have a total lack of insulin (type 1 diabetes) or they have too little insulin or cannot use insulin effectively (type 2 diabetes). Those with Type 1 are either born with it or they develop it at a very young age. Type 2 is also referred to as adult onset diabetes because they usually develop it well into adulthood.

Contrary to what many people think, diabetes isn't just caused from eating too many sweets. In fact, diabetes is more commonly caused from eating too many calories all together paired with little or no physical activity. Here are some risk factors for type 2 diabetes:

- High blood pressure
- High blood triglyceride (fat) levels
- Gestational diabetes or giving birth to a baby weighing more than 9 pounds
- **High-fat and carbohydrate diet**
- High alcohol intake
- **Sedentary lifestyle**
- **Obesity or being overweight**
- Ethnicity: Certain groups, such as African Americans, Native Americans, Hispanic Americans, and Asian Americans, have a greater risk of developing type 2 diabetes than non-Hispanic whites.
- Aging: Increasing age is a significant risk factor for type 2 diabetes. The risk of developing type 2 diabetes begins to rise significantly at about age 45, and rises considerably after age 65.

You Ate What???

Keep up the good work and when you get some time, start taking a look back at some of your food journals from the earlier rounds and see where you're improving.

Food Journal

Time of meal 1 - _________

Food eaten- ____

Drink - _________________________

Carbohydrates		**Protein**		**Fat**	
Total crab grams -		Total protein grams -		Total fat grams -	
Total fiber grams -		Total protein calories -		Total fat calories	
Total sugar grams -				Total saturated	
Total complex grams -				Total unsaturated -	
Total carb calories -					
Percentage of meal -	%	Percentage of meal -	%	Percentage of meal -	%

Total calories of meal - **cal**
Total ounces of water with meal - **ounces**
Total sodium of meal - **mgs**

Time of meal 2 - ________

Food eaten- ____

Drink - ______________________

Carbohydrates		**Protein**		**Fat**	
Total crab grams -		Total protein grams -		Total fat grams -	
Total fiber grams -		Total protein calories -		Total fat calories	
Total sugar grams -				Total saturated	
Total complex grams -				Total unsaturated -	
Total carb calories -					
Percentage of meal -	%	Percentage of meal -	%	Percentage of meal -	%

Total calories of meal - **cal**
Total ounces of water with meal - **ounces**
Total sodium of meal - **mgs**

Time of meal 3 (Lunch) - ________

Food eaten- ____

Drink - ______________________

Carbohydrates		**Protein**		**Fat**	
Total crab grams -		Total protein grams -		Total fat grams -	
Total fiber grams -		Total protein calories -		Total fat calories	
Total sugar grams -				Total saturated	
Total complex grams -				Total unsaturated -	
Total carb calories -					
Percentage of meal -	%	Percentage of meal -	%	Percentage of meal -	%

Total calories of meal - **cal**
Total ounces of water with meal - **ounces**
Total sodium of meal - **mgs**

Time of meal 4 - ________

Food eaten- ____

Drink - ______________________

Carbohydrates	**Protein**	**Fat**
Total crab grams -	Total protein grams -	Total fat grams -
Total fiber grams -	Total protein calories -	Total fat calories
Total sugar grams -		Total saturated
Total complex grams -		Total unsaturated -
Total carb calories -		
Percentage of meal - %	Percentage of meal - %	Percentage of meal - %

Total calories of meal - cal
Total ounces of water with meal - ounces
Total sodium of meal - mgs

Time of meal 5 - _________

Food eaten- ____

Drink - ________________________

Carbohydrates	**Protein**	**Fat**
Total crab grams -	Total protein grams -	Total fat grams -
Total fiber grams -	Total protein calories -	Total fat calories
Total sugar grams -		Total saturated
Total complex grams -		Total unsaturated -
Total carb calories -		
Percentage of meal - %	Percentage of meal - %	Percentage of meal - %

Total calories of meal - cal
Total ounces of water with meal - ounces
Total sodium of meal - mgs

Total ounces of water with meals - ounces
Total ounces of water outside meals - ounces
Total ounces of water today - ounces
Total sodium today - mgs

Another great day for you; now go rest up and get ready for your back and bicep day tomorrow. Don't forget to look at your workout for tomorrow so you'll know what's coming; it's going to be a good one.

Round 10 - Day 5

Hey Champ! How did you sleep last night? By the way; what's for breakfast? Did you make enough for me? Coming up in the next round were going to start taking a closer look at each of your meals to make sure you getting the right kinds of foods and the right amount of calories at the right times.

That One Thing

On Day 1 of this round, you were to think of a way you can give back by volunteering somewhere for a great cause. Today I want you to think of one person you can get to go with you and ask them within the next three days. Tell them they have to go with you because this book says so.

Seeing I to Eye

Take 5-10 minutes today and think about a big change you've made from using 12 Rounds. Once you've got it in your head, visualize yourself making this change with the ways you use it in your daily life.

Your Workout – See your workout log for today's workout.

And the Heart Says…

Tonight after dinner and when you've been relaxing for about an hour, take and record a heart rate. Start looking back at your earlier rounds and see what's changed with your heart rates.

Evening resting HR ______ Time taken ______

Cleaning Your Plate

What exactly is an "empty calorie"?

Foods with **empty calories** have lots of calories but very few nutrients like vitamins and minerals. "Convenience foods," like packaged snacks, chips, and sodas, processed lunch meats, dairy products made from whole milk, crackers, french fries, and sugary treats are common sources of empty calories and should be avoided.

Eating empty calories is like putting a cheap, low grade and dirty fuel in your vehicle and expecting it to run great. Do you think airplanes use dirty fuel?

You Ate What???

It is very common for people to almost remove all fat from their diets when they want to lose weight. You know by now that this is not the way to do it. While you're making sure you're not eating too much fat calories, make sure you're getting enough as well. Shoot for 30% of your daily calories to be from good unsaturated fat; with a little saturated fat as well.

Food Journal

Time of meal 1 - _________

Food eaten- ____

Drink - ________________________

Carbohydrates	**Protein**	**Fat**
Total crab grams -	Total protein grams -	Total fat grams -
Total fiber grams -	Total protein calories -	Total fat calories
Total sugar grams -		Total saturated
Total complex grams -		Total unsaturated -
Total carb calories -		
Percentage of meal - %	Percentage of meal - %	Percentage of meal - %

Total calories of meal - cal
Total ounces of water with meal - ounces
Total sodium of meal - mgs

Time of meal 2 - _________

Food eaten- ____

Drink - ________________________

Carbohydrates		**Protein**		**Fat**	
Total crab grams -		Total protein grams -		Total fat grams -	
Total fiber grams -		Total protein calories -		Total fat calories	
Total sugar grams -				Total saturated	
Total complex grams -				Total unsaturated -	
Total carb calories -					
Percentage of meal -	%	Percentage of meal -	%	Percentage of meal -	%

Total calories of meal - **cal**
Total ounces of water with meal - **ounces**
Total sodium of meal - **mgs**

Time of meal 3 (Lunch) - _________

Food eaten- ____

Drink - ________________________

Carbohydrates		**Protein**		**Fat**	
Total crab grams -		Total protein grams -		Total fat grams -	
Total fiber grams -		Total protein calories -		Total fat calories	
Total sugar grams -				Total saturated	
Total complex grams -				Total unsaturated -	
Total carb calories -					
Percentage of meal -	%	Percentage of meal -	%	Percentage of meal -	%

Total calories of meal - **cal**
Total ounces of water with meal - **ounces**
Total sodium of meal - **mgs**

Time of meal 4 - _________

Food eaten- ____

Drink - ________________________

Carbohydrates		**Protein**		**Fat**	
Total crab grams -		Total protein grams -		Total fat grams -	
Total fiber grams -		Total protein calories -		Total fat calories	
Total sugar grams -				Total saturated	
Total complex grams -				Total unsaturated -	
Total carb calories -					
Percentage of meal -	%	Percentage of meal -	%	Percentage of meal -	%

Total calories of meal - **cal**
Total ounces of water with meal - **ounces**
Total sodium of meal - **mgs**

Time of meal 5 - ________

Food eaten- ____

Drink - ________________________

Carbohydrates		**Protein**		**Fat**	
Total crab grams -		Total protein grams -		Total fat grams -	
Total fiber grams -		Total protein calories -		Total fat calories	
Total sugar grams -				Total saturated	
Total complex grams -				Total unsaturated -	
Total carb calories -					
Percentage of meal -	%	Percentage of meal -	%	Percentage of meal -	%

Total calories of meal - **cal**
Total ounces of water with meal - **ounces**
Total sodium of meal - **mgs**

Total ounces of water with meals - **ounces**
Total ounces of water during workout - **ounces**
Total ounces of water outside meals - **ounces**
Total ounces of water today - **ounces**
Total sodium today - **mgs**

That's five days in the bag with two more to go. Are you ready for core and cardio tomorrow? I guess we'll soon find out.

Round 10 - Day 6

Here we go: Day 6! The one thing I want to remind you of before you get started with your core and cardio workout today is to make sure you're going slowly on your core exercises. Make sure you're taking 4-5 seconds as well as pausing at the top and bottom of every single rep you do; this is what makes this program work so well. Now go get after it!

Which Way You Headed?

On Day 2 you were to help someone set a goal about something other than their fitness and on Day 4 you were to help someone set a goal about their fitness. Today, help that same person or a new person set a goal about their career. A great way to get the ball rolling is to show them your goals with 12 Rounds. Go ahead; show off a little.

Upper Management

On Day 1 you were to find a place where you can volunteer and make a plan to do so. If you haven't found a spot to volunteer, do that today and mark it in your calendar. Don't let this slip away because wherever you end up helping out, it will make you feel amazing for doing it, and you'll more than likely make some new friends too.

Seeing I to Eye

Think back to one of the greatest memories you have of being with family or friends like during the holidays, a vacation, someone's birthday, a wedding, or any other time where you had a blast. Go get in that quiet place, clear your head, and take yourself right back to that time and enjoy it all over again.

Your Workout – See your workout log for today's workout.

And the Heart Says…

At some point this evening when you are relaxed, take another heart rate and record it here.

Post workout evening HR ______ Time taken __________

Cleaning Your Plate

How can drinking alcohol cause me to gain weight?

It's really very simple. Alcohol has calories just like food and if you do drink alcohol, you need to count these calories juts like to the food you eat. Most of the calories in alcohol are in the form of carbohydrates because many types of alcohol are made from grains and potatoes so be sure to take count of these in your food journal.

Another way alcohol causes weight gain is its ability to inhibit leptin; the hormone that promotes a feeling of fullness. In addition to blocking the signal from your body that you're full, alcohol can impair your judgment where you eat too much food and bad food. Those late night drive through fast food places are there for a reason. It's been a while, but I am guilty of doing it too.

You Ate What???

Keep working toward getting those ratios where you want them. I know it's a full time job, but the benefits of a lifetime are coming from you doing this so keep at it. Watch that sodium!

Food Journal

Time of meal 1 - _________

Food eaten- ____

Drink - ________________________

Carbohydrates		**Protein**		**Fat**	
Total crab grams -		Total protein grams -		Total fat grams -	
Total fiber grams -		Total protein calories -		Total fat calories	
Total sugar grams -				Total saturated	
Total complex grams -				Total unsaturated -	
Total carb calories -					
Percentage of meal -	%	Percentage of meal -	%	Percentage of meal -	%

Total calories of meal - cal
Total ounces of water with meal - ounces
Total sodium of meal - mgs

Time of meal 2 - _________

Food eaten- ____

Drink - ________________________

Carbohydrates	**Protein**	**Fat**
Total crab grams -	Total protein grams -	Total fat grams -
Total fiber grams -	Total protein calories -	Total fat calories
Total sugar grams -		Total saturated
Total complex grams -		Total unsaturated -
Total carb calories -		
Percentage of meal - %	Percentage of meal - %	Percentage of meal - %

Total calories of meal - cal
Total ounces of water with meal - ounces
Total sodium of meal - mgs

Time of meal 3 (Lunch) - _________

Food eaten- ____

Drink - ________________________

Carbohydrates	**Protein**	**Fat**
Total crab grams -	Total protein grams -	Total fat grams -
Total fiber grams -	Total protein calories -	Total fat calories
Total sugar grams -		Total saturated
Total complex grams -		Total unsaturated -
Total carb calories -		
Percentage of meal - %	Percentage of meal - %	Percentage of meal - %

Total calories of meal - cal
Total ounces of water with meal - ounces
Total sodium of meal - mgs

Time of meal 4 - _________

Food eaten- ____

Drink - ________________________

Carbohydrates	**Protein**	**Fat**
Total crab grams -	Total protein grams -	Total fat grams -
Total fiber grams -	Total protein calories -	Total fat calories
Total sugar grams -		Total saturated
Total complex grams -		Total unsaturated -
Total carb calories -		
Percentage of meal - %	Percentage of meal - %	Percentage of meal - %

Total calories of meal - cal
Total ounces of water with meal - ounces
Total sodium of meal - mgs

Time of meal 5 - _________

Food eaten- ____

Drink - ________________________

Carbohydrates	**Protein**	**Fat**
Total crab grams -	Total protein grams -	Total fat grams -
Total fiber grams -	Total protein calories -	Total fat calories
Total sugar grams -		Total saturated
Total complex grams -		Total unsaturated -
Total carb calories -		
Percentage of meal - %	Percentage of meal - %	Percentage of meal - %

Total calories of meal - cal
Total ounces of water with meal - ounces
Total sodium of meal - mgs

Total ounces of water with meals - ounces
Total ounces of water during workout - ounces
Total ounces of water outside meals - ounces
Total ounces of water today - ounces
Total sodium today - mgs

How are you doing with Round 10? I told you it would be different but I wouldn't have put it in here if it wasn't important. Keep smiling and making your way through 12 Rounds; you're headed toward your best self yet!

Round 10- Day 7

One more day of Round 10 and then it's off to the last two rounds. Take a day off today and enjoy the progress you've made to this point. I'll see you tomorrow for the start of Round 11!

I took this heart rate when I was…____

Day 7 HR ______ Time taken _______

Food Journal

Time of meal 1 - _________

Food eaten- ____

Drink - _________________________

Carbohydrates	**Protein**	**Fat**
Total crab grams -	Total protein grams -	Total fat grams -
Total fiber grams -	Total protein calories -	Total fat calories
Total sugar grams -		Total saturated
Total complex grams -		Total unsaturated -
Total carb calories -		
Percentage of meal - %	Percentage of meal - %	Percentage of meal - %

Total calories of meal - cal
Total ounces of water with meal - ounces
Total sodium of meal - mgs

Time of meal 2 - _________

Food eaten- ____

Drink - ________________________

Carbohydrates		**Protein**		**Fat**	
Total crab grams -		Total protein grams -		Total fat grams -	
Total fiber grams -		Total protein calories -		Total fat calories	
Total sugar grams -				Total saturated	
Total complex grams -				Total unsaturated -	
Total carb calories -					
Percentage of meal -	%	Percentage of meal -	%	Percentage of meal -	%

Total calories of meal - **cal**
Total ounces of water with meal - **ounces**
Total sodium of meal - **mgs**

Time of meal 3 (Lunch) - _________

Food eaten- ____

Drink - ________________________

Carbohydrates		**Protein**		**Fat**	
Total crab grams -		Total protein grams -		Total fat grams -	
Total fiber grams -		Total protein calories -		Total fat calories	
Total sugar grams -				Total saturated	
Total complex grams -				Total unsaturated -	
Total carb calories -					
Percentage of meal -	%	Percentage of meal -	%	Percentage of meal -	%

Total calories of meal - **cal**
Total ounces of water with meal - **ounces**
Total sodium of meal - **mgs**

Time of meal 4 - _________

Food eaten- ____

Drink - ________________________

Carbohydrates		**Protein**		**Fat**	
Total crab grams -		Total protein grams -		Total fat grams -	
Total fiber grams -		Total protein calories -		Total fat calories	
Total sugar grams -				Total saturated	
Total complex grams -				Total unsaturated -	
Total carb calories -					
Percentage of meal -	%	Percentage of meal -	%	Percentage of meal -	%

Total calories of meal - **cal**
Total ounces of water with meal - **ounces**
Total sodium of meal - **mgs**

Time of meal 5 - _________

Food eaten- ____

Drink - ________________________

Carbohydrates		**Protein**		**Fat**	
Total crab grams -		Total protein grams -		Total fat grams -	
Total fiber grams -		Total protein calories -		Total fat calories	
Total sugar grams -				Total saturated	
Total complex grams -				Total unsaturated -	
Total carb calories -					
Percentage of meal -	%	Percentage of meal -	%	Percentage of meal -	%

Total calories of meal - **cal**
Total ounces of water with meal - **ounces**
Total sodium of meal - **mgs**

Total ounces of water with meals - **ounces**
Total ounces of water outside meals - **ounces**
Total ounces of water today - **ounces**
Total sodium today - **mgs**

Round 11 – Strength in Numbers

Day 1

To this point in 12 Rounds, you have built something amazing and these next two rounds are all about finishing it off with a bang! Let's make these last 14 days the best one's yet by staying strong, staying committed, and putting yourself in a place you've never been before. I know you're ready; let's go all out!

"When your support, encouragement, and motivation come from many, the top of the mountain you're climbing starts to look more like a hill." **Bobby Whisnand**

It Happened Just Like This!

About three years ago I started an exercise class called "It's All Heart" and something happened within this class I never expected. Every Wednesday night we would spend the first half of the class talking about everyone's goals. I had expected this would be the night where I would have the least amount of people show up, but it turned out to be the opposite. On this night, I would have 2-3 times more people show up than on any other night. One night I asked the class why so many of them show up for the Wednesday class and not the others. They all answered my question very quickly by saying, "This is the one place where we can get back on track no matter what happens during the week. This is where we can reset, get support to reach our goals, and get back on track with everything in our lives, not just exercise and eating right."

You may know this to be true, but the more support you have, the better chance you have at reaching your goals and improving your life. Don't be afraid to share your goals with other people; they might just have the same goals as you, and that my friend is the making of a new partner and a new friend.

That One Thing

Think about one part of your life other than exercise and eating well which you have improved by doing 12 Rounds. Once you have it, write it down here and share it with someone.

One part of my life other than exercise and eating well which I have improved with 12 Rounds is…

____

Seeing I to Eye

In Round 2 I asked you to visualize yourself doing something in which you have very little confidence. Take 5-6 minutes today and visualize it again except this time, make sure you can see many people standing around applauding and cheering as you're doing it.

Your Workout – See your workout log for today's workout

And the Heart Says…

After you take this heart rate, take a look back at your heart rates during the first two rounds and see what the difference is.

Pre Sleep HR - ______ Time taken ________

Cleaning Your Plate

Be very careful about those food packaging labels like ***"No Sugar Added", "Low Sodium", and "1/3 Less Calories"***. When it comes to food packaging, companies will do their best to catch your eye with hugely printed wording on labels like the ones I just listed. The only true way to know if the food in any package is healthy, low sugar, and low sodium, is to look at the ingredients and read the nutrition labels on the back. Regardless of what those big print letters say, the truth lies in the nutrition label so don't get suckered in with their marketing ploys. You're smarter than that, and you know exactly what to look for now.

You Ate What???

You've spent a lot of time filling out these food journals and it's time to make the most of them. There are two main things I want you to look for in your journals this week: If you're trying to lose body weight and body fat, keep your food ratios at 30% carbs/40% protein/ 30% fat as well as removing your carbohydrates from your last two meals with the exception of green vegetables. On the other hand, if you're trying to gain weight, keep your food ratios at 40% carbs/30% protein/30% fat and increase your total caloric intake across each day.

Food Journal

Time of meal 1 - _________

Food eaten- ____

Drink - ________________________

Carbohydrates	**Protein**	**Fat**
Total crab grams -	Total protein grams -	Total fat grams -
Total fiber grams -	Total protein calories -	Total fat calories
Total sugar grams -		Total saturated
Total complex grams -		Total unsaturated -
Total carb calories -		
Percentage of meal - %	Percentage of meal - %	Percentage of meal - %

Total calories of meal - cal
Total ounces of water with meal - ounces
Total sodium of meal - mgs

Time of meal 2 - _________

Food eaten- ____

Drink - ________________________

Carbohydrates	**Protein**	**Fat**
Total crab grams -	Total protein grams -	Total fat grams -
Total fiber grams -	Total protein calories -	Total fat calories
Total sugar grams -		Total saturated
Total complex grams -		Total unsaturated -
Total carb calories -		
Percentage of meal - %	Percentage of meal - %	Percentage of meal - %

Total calories of meal - cal
Total ounces of water with meal - ounces
Total sodium of meal - mgs

Time of meal 3 (Lunch) - _________

Food eaten- ____

Drink - ________________________

Carbohydrates		**Protein**		**Fat**	
Total crab grams -		Total protein grams -		Total fat grams -	
Total fiber grams -		Total protein calories -		Total fat calories	
Total sugar grams -				Total saturated	
Total complex grams -				Total unsaturated -	
Total carb calories -					
Percentage of meal -	%	Percentage of meal -	%	Percentage of meal -	%

Total calories of meal - **cal**
Total ounces of water with meal - **ounces**
Total sodium of meal - **mgs**

Time of meal 4 - _________

Food eaten- ____

Drink - ________________________

Carbohydrates		**Protein**		**Fat**	
Total crab grams -		Total protein grams -		Total fat grams -	
Total fiber grams -		Total protein calories -		Total fat calories	
Total sugar grams -				Total saturated	
Total complex grams -				Total unsaturated -	
Total carb calories -					
Percentage of meal -	%	Percentage of meal -	%	Percentage of meal -	%

Total calories of meal - **cal**
Total ounces of water with meal - **ounces**
Total sodium of meal - **mgs**

Time of meal 5 - _________

Food eaten- ____

Drink - ________________________

Carbohydrates		**Protein**		**Fat**	
Total crab grams -		Total protein grams -		Total fat grams -	
Total fiber grams -		Total protein calories -		Total fat calories	
Total sugar grams -				Total saturated	
Total complex grams -				Total unsaturated -	
Total carb calories -					
Percentage of meal -	%	Percentage of meal -	%	Percentage of meal -	%

Total calories of meal - **cal**
Total ounces of water with meal - **ounces**
Total sodium of meal - **mgs**

Total ounces of water with meals - ounces
Total ounces of water during workout - ounces
Total ounces of water outside meals - ounces
Total ounces of water today - ounces
Total sodium today - mgs

That's the way to start Round 11: Great job! Take a close look at your workout coming up tomorrow, get some good clean food in your body, and put that mind in a good place before you go to sleep. I'll see you tomorrow for Day 2.

Round 11 - Day 2

I hope you're ready for a tough core workout today. I'm going to split your core and cardio away from each other so you can do all of your core exercises without stopping. I bet that just made your day, right? Let's do it!

Which Way You Headed?

Last week I gave you a break on writing your goals but being this is the second to the last week, we're going to ramp it up.

Write your three long term goals about something other than your fitness and while you're at it, write down two things you can do over the next two weeks to reach each goal.

Goal 1 - ____

The first thing I can do over the next two weeks to reach this goal is...

____

The second thing I can do over the next two weeks to reach this goal is...

____

Goal 2 - ____

The first thing I can do over the next two weeks to reach this goal is...

____

The second thing I can do over the next two weeks to reach this goal is...

____

Goal 3 - ____

The first thing I can do over the next two weeks to reach this goal is...

____

The second thing I can do over the next two weeks to reach this goal is...

____

Seeing I to Eye

If you could have any occupation you wanted, what would it be? After you decide what it is, take 5-6 minutes today and visualize yourself doing it and enjoying it. I can't tell you mine; you'd just laugh at me.

Upper Management

Not all stress is bad, but it can turn bad very quickly if you do not get rid of it. One way to get rid of stress is to talk to someone about it. Get with that person with whom you are comfortable and talk about a stress you have. I know this can be hard to do, but they will appreciate the fact that you asked them to listen and it will make you feel tons better.

Your Workout – See your workout log for today's workout.

Cleaning Your Plate

What is Ketosis?

Ketosis is a word you'll probably see when you're looking for information on diabetes or weight loss. Ketosis is a normal metabolic process, something your body does to keep working. When it doesn't have enough carbohydrates from food for your cells to burn for energy, it burns fat instead. As part of this process, it makes ketones.

If you're healthy and eating a balanced diet, your body controls how much fat it burns, and you don't normally make or use ketones. But when you cut way back on your calories or carbs, your body will switch to ketosis for energy. For people with uncontrolled diabetes, ketosis is a sign of not using enough insulin.

Ketosis can become dangerous when ketones build up. High levels lead to dehydration and change the chemical balance of your blood so you don't want to restrict your body of calories and carbohydrates to the point where ketones are building to unhealthy levels. This is exactly why I say to keep some level of complex carbs in your diet no matter what your body weight goals are.

You Ate What???

What percentage of carbohydrates are you coming up with on average in your daily food journals? Make sure you keep track of this because as I said very early on in 12 Rounds, carbohydrate intake is a big key to maintaining a healthy body weight. Your carbohydrate percentage should be between 30-40% of your diet.

Food Journal

Time of meal 1 - _________

Food eaten- ____

Drink - ________________________

Carbohydrates		**Protein**		**Fat**	
Total crab grams -		Total protein grams -		Total fat grams -	
Total fiber grams -		Total protein calories -		Total fat calories	
Total sugar grams -				Total saturated	
Total complex grams -				Total unsaturated -	
Total carb calories -					
Percentage of meal -	%	Percentage of meal -	%	Percentage of meal -	%

Total calories of meal - **cal**
Total ounces of water with meal - **ounces**
Total sodium of meal - **mgs**

Time of meal 2 - _________

Food eaten- ____

Drink - ________________________

Carbohydrates		**Protein**		**Fat**	
Total crab grams -		Total protein grams -		Total fat grams -	
Total fiber grams -		Total protein calories -		Total fat calories	
Total sugar grams -				Total saturated	
Total complex grams -				Total unsaturated -	
Total carb calories -					
Percentage of meal -	%	Percentage of meal -	%	Percentage of meal -	%

Total calories of meal - **cal**
Total ounces of water with meal - **ounces**
Total sodium of meal - **mgs**

Time of meal 3 (Lunch) - _________

Food eaten- ____

Drink - ________________________

Carbohydrates		**Protein**		**Fat**	
Total crab grams -		Total protein grams -		Total fat grams -	
Total fiber grams -		Total protein calories -		Total fat calories	
Total sugar grams -				Total saturated	
Total complex grams -				Total unsaturated -	
Total carb calories -					
Percentage of meal -	%	Percentage of meal -	%	Percentage of meal -	%

Total calories of meal - **cal**
Total ounces of water with meal - **ounces**
Total sodium of meal - **mgs**

Time of meal 4 - ________

Food eaten- ____

Drink - ________________________

Carbohydrates		**Protein**		**Fat**	
Total crab grams -		Total protein grams -		Total fat grams -	
Total fiber grams -		Total protein calories -		Total fat calories	
Total sugar grams -				Total saturated	
Total complex grams -				Total unsaturated -	
Total carb calories -					
Percentage of meal -	%	Percentage of meal -	%	Percentage of meal -	%

Total calories of meal - **cal**
Total ounces of water with meal - **ounces**
Total sodium of meal - **mgs**

Time of meal 5 - ________

Food eaten- ____

Drink - ________________________

Carbohydrates		**Protein**		**Fat**	
Total crab grams -		Total protein grams -		Total fat grams -	
Total fiber grams -		Total protein calories -		Total fat calories	
Total sugar grams -				Total saturated	
Total complex grams -				Total unsaturated -	
Total carb calories -					
Percentage of meal -	%	Percentage of meal -	%	Percentage of meal -	%

Total calories of meal - **cal**
Total ounces of water with meal - **ounces**
Total sodium of meal - **mgs**

Total ounces of water with meals - **ounces**
Total ounces of water during workout - **ounces**
Total ounces of water outside meals - **ounces**
Total ounces of water today - **ounces**
Total sodium today - **mgs**

And The Heart Says…

At some point in the middle of your day, take a heart rate and record it here. Start taking a look back through your earlier rounds and see what changes are happening with your heart rates.

Afternoon HR-________ Time taken - _______

I know I've asked you this a hundred times by now but are you making sure you are drinking enough water during your days? I think you should shoot for 90-100 ounces a day, especially if you are sticking to the exercise parts of 12 Rounds. Don't forget to drink 10-12 ounces of water as soon as you get up in the morning too.

Round 11 – Day 3

Good morning Champ! Did you have any good dreams last night? I did, but I'm not going to tell you what they were because you will only make fun of me. Make sure you look at the Appendix in the back of your workout journal before you work out today so you can see what your weights should look like. I'm going to go get warmed up because I've got another great leg workout for you today.

That One Thing

Think about one part of your exercise and eating which you have improved by doing 12 Rounds. Once you have it, write it down here and go share it with someone.

One part of my exercise and eating which I have improved with 12 Rounds is...

Seeing I to Eye

Think about an over the top daredevil activity you have always wanted to try like skydiving, zip lining, demolition derby, tubing down the mountain on snow, or anything else you can think of. Once you've got it figured out, take 5-6 minutes visualizing yourself doing it and be sure to add sounds, colors, noises, and other people. Go ahead and let it fly. By the way, mine is...never mind.

Your Workout – See your workout log for today's workout

And the Heart Says...

While you're at work today and sitting at your desk, take a heart rate and write it down here. Make sure you've been sitting for at least 5 minutes before you take it.

Resting HR - ______ Time Taken - ________

Cleaning Your Plate

What is Creatine and should you take it?

Creatine is a nitrogenous organic acid produced in the liver that helps supply energy to cells all over the body - particularly muscle cells. It is made out of three amino acids: L-arginine, glycine, and L-methionine. It is widely used as a strength, energy, and performance enhancing supplement by many athletes, but just as much or more so by those who weight train and body build.

Now, should you use it or not? It's really up to you and if you do so, let your doctor know so they can give you some precautions about taking creatine. I for one believe in its effectiveness and I use it on a regular basis.

You Ate What???

Use the next week and a half to really clean up your diet if you already haven't. Get those 4-5 meals in a every day, eat the right ratio of foods, keep your sodium low, and drink plenty of water throughout your day. I'm counting on you!

Food Journal

Time of meal 1 - _________

Food eaten- ____

Drink - ________________________

Carbohydrates		**Protein**		**Fat**	
Total crab grams -		Total protein grams -		Total fat grams -	
Total fiber grams -		Total protein calories -		Total fat calories	
Total sugar grams -				Total saturated	
Total complex grams -				Total unsaturated -	
Total carb calories -					
Percentage of meal -	%	Percentage of meal -	%	Percentage of meal -	%

Total calories of meal - **cal**
Total ounces of water with meal - **ounces**
Total sodium of meal - **mgs**

Time of meal 2 - _________

Food eaten- ____

Drink - ________________________

Carbohydrates		**Protein**		**Fat**	
Total crab grams -		Total protein grams -		Total fat grams -	
Total fiber grams -		Total protein calories -		Total fat calories	
Total sugar grams -				Total saturated	
Total complex grams -				Total unsaturated -	
Total carb calories -					
Percentage of meal -	%	Percentage of meal -	%	Percentage of meal -	%

Total calories of meal - **cal**
Total ounces of water with meal - **ounces**
Total sodium of meal - **mgs**

Time of meal 3 (Lunch) - _________

Food eaten- ____

Drink - ________________________

Carbohydrates		**Protein**		**Fat**	
Total crab grams -		Total protein grams -		Total fat grams -	
Total fiber grams -		Total protein calories -		Total fat calories	
Total sugar grams -				Total saturated	
Total complex grams -				Total unsaturated -	
Total carb calories -					
Percentage of meal -	%	Percentage of meal -	%	Percentage of meal -	%

Total calories of meal - **cal**
Total ounces of water with meal - **ounces**
Total sodium of meal - **mgs**

Time of meal 4 - _________

Food eaten- ____

Drink - ________________________

Carbohydrates	**Protein**	**Fat**
Total crab grams -	Total protein grams -	Total fat grams -
Total fiber grams -	Total protein calories -	Total fat calories
Total sugar grams -		Total saturated
Total complex grams -		Total unsaturated -
Total carb calories -		
Percentage of meal - %	Percentage of meal - %	Percentage of meal - %

Total calories of meal - cal
Total ounces of water with meal - ounces
Total sodium of meal - mgs

Time of meal 5 - _________

Food eaten- ____

Drink - ________________________

Carbohydrates	**Protein**	**Fat**
Total crab grams -	Total protein grams -	Total fat grams -
Total fiber grams -	Total protein calories -	Total fat calories
Total sugar grams -		Total saturated
Total complex grams -		Total unsaturated -
Total carb calories -		
Percentage of meal - %	Percentage of meal - %	Percentage of meal - %

Total calories of meal - cal
Total ounces of water with meal - ounces
Total sodium of meal - mgs

Total ounces of water with meals - ounces
Total ounces of water during workout - ounces
Total ounces of water outside meals - ounces
Total ounces of water today - ounces
Total sodium today - mgs

That was a great leg day for you; now go do what you need to do to let them recuperate. That means good food, good sleep, and good thoughts. I'll see you tomorrow!

Round 11 - Day 4

How's that body feel today? One thing I tell every single person that works out is to take a day off after working out their legs. Your entire body needs more recuperation after leg day so make sure you give it what it needs and it all starts with a day off. But that doesn't mean you can't work your brain a little bit, right?

"There are lots of people, relationships, and companies that have communication problems. That's because some only talk and others only listen which leads to nobody really sharing anything."

Bobby Whisnand

It Happened Just Like This!

I was presenting for an IT company last year and to get things going, I asked a gentleman in the front what was one of his current goals in his life. He said, "To save $50,000 for my daughter's wedding next year." I responded by saying "better you than me", and once every one stopped laughing, I told him my goal was to give 24 keynote speeches over the next year. I jumped down from the stage, walked over the gentleman, and after I shook his hand, I asked the entire audience to pair up with a person next to them and tell each other one goal they currently have. I spent the next minute talking with this man and then returned to the stage to find the entire audience in conversation. I had to actually call their attention back to me and then I asked them, "How long has it been since you guys communicated like that? Also, how many of you have the same goals?" The rest of my presentation was awesome, and after it was over, a lady from upper management came up to me and said, "For a communications company, you'd think we talked more but we don't. This is the most I have ever seen this company communicate at once; thanks for opening our minds and our mouths."

Sharing your goals with others creates three things; instant encouragement, another point of view, and quite possibly some of the best advice you've ever had. Either way; it's a win-win situation.

Which Way You Headed?

Write your three long term goals about your fitness, and while you're at it, write down two things you can do over the next two weeks to reach each goal.

Goal 1 - ____

The first thing I can do over the next two weeks to reach this goal is…

____

The second thing I can do over the next two weeks to reach this goal is…

____

Goal 2 - ____

The first thing I can do over the next two weeks to reach this goal is…

____

The second thing I can do over the next two weeks to reach this goal is…

____

Goal 3 - ____

The first thing I can do over the next two weeks to reach this goal is…

____

The second thing I can do over the next two weeks to reach this goal is…

____

Seeing I to Eye

Have you ever had a dream where you could fly? I have, and I think it's awesome! And if I wake up, I try to go back to sleep and fly some more but it doesn't work like that. However, as good as you are at visualizing now, you can fly whenever and wherever you want. Take 5-6 minutes today, clear your mind, and fly through the mountains, the city, in the clouds, in space, or wherever you want. Go ahead; they're your wings and you should use them.

Upper Management

On Day 2 you were to get with someone and tell them about a stress you have in your life. Today, get with that person and ask them if they have a stress they would like share with you. If they have nothing to share at the time, let them know they can always give you a ring to talk about it.

No Workout Today!

And the Heart Says…

Take at least one heart rate today whenever you want. Just make sure you write down when and under what circumstances you took it.

Today I took my heart rate when I was… __________________________________

Day 4 HR - ______ Time taken - ________

Cleaning Your Plate

If I eat 4-5 meals a day, do they all have to be full meals?

We talked about this earlier in 12 Rounds but I wanted to talk about it a little more. The answer is no; an ideal eating plan would have three regular meals and two smaller meals in between for snacks. For example: For my 2nd meal which is a snack in between breakfast and lunch, I might have a 20-30 gram protein drink with a piece of fruit and maybe some nuts. For my 4th meal which is a snack in between lunch and dinner, I might eat the same things I did for my 2nd meal or something different like a few boiled egg whites, a piece of fruit, and some more nuts. Either way; keep your calories spread throughout the day and keep the larger concentration of calories for breakfast and lunch.

You Ate What???

Keep up the good work on your food journal and when you get some time, start taking a look back at some of your food journals from the earlier rounds and see where you're improving.

Food Journal

Time of meal 1 - _________

Food eaten- ____

Drink - ________________________

Carbohydrates		**Protein**		**Fat**	
Total crab grams -		Total protein grams -		Total fat grams -	
Total fiber grams -		Total protein calories -		Total fat calories	
Total sugar grams -				Total saturated	
Total complex grams -				Total unsaturated -	
Total carb calories -					
Percentage of meal -	%	Percentage of meal -	%	Percentage of meal -	%

Total calories of meal - **cal**
Total ounces of water with meal - **ounces**
Total sodium of meal - **mgs**

Time of meal 2 - _________

Food eaten- ____

Drink - ________________________

Carbohydrates		**Protein**		**Fat**	
Total crab grams -		Total protein grams -		Total fat grams -	
Total fiber grams -		Total protein calories -		Total fat calories	
Total sugar grams -				Total saturated	
Total complex grams -				Total unsaturated -	
Total carb calories -					
Percentage of meal -	%	Percentage of meal -	%	Percentage of meal -	%

Total calories of meal - **cal**
Total ounces of water with meal - **ounces**
Total sodium of meal - **mgs**

Time of meal 3 (Lunch) ________

Food eaten- ____

Drink - ________________________

Carbohydrates		**Protein**		**Fat**	
Total crab grams -		Total protein grams -		Total fat grams -	
Total fiber grams -		Total protein calories -		Total fat calories	
Total sugar grams -				Total saturated	
Total complex grams -				Total unsaturated -	
Total carb calories -					
Percentage of meal -	%	Percentage of meal -	%	Percentage of meal -	%

Total calories of meal - **cal**
Total ounces of water with meal - **ounces**
Total sodium of meal - **mgs**

Time of meal 4 - _________

Food eaten- ____

Drink - ________________________

Carbohydrates		**Protein**		**Fat**	
Total crab grams -		Total protein grams -		Total fat grams -	
Total fiber grams -		Total protein calories -		Total fat calories	
Total sugar grams -				Total saturated	
Total complex grams -				Total unsaturated -	
Total carb calories -					
Percentage of meal -	%	Percentage of meal -	%	Percentage of meal -	%

Total calories of meal - **cal**
Total ounces of water with meal - **ounces**
Total sodium of meal - **mgs**

Time of meal 5 - _________

Food eaten- ____

Drink - ________________________

Carbohydrates		**Protein**		**Fat**	
Total crab grams -		Total protein grams -		Total fat grams -	
Total fiber grams -		Total protein calories -		Total fat calories	
Total sugar grams -				Total saturated	
Total complex grams -				Total unsaturated -	
Total carb calories -					
Percentage of meal -	%	Percentage of meal -	%	Percentage of meal -	%

Total calories of meal - **cal**
Total ounces of water with meal - **ounces**
Total sodium of meal - **mgs**

Total ounces of water with meals - **ounces**
Total ounces of water outside meals - **ounces**
Total ounces of water today - **ounces**
Total sodium today - **mgs**

I guess it's time for you to end your day but don't forget to take some time to look over tomorrow's workout in your workout journal. If you're not pre-marking your weights for the next day's workout, give it a shot and see how it saves you time. Okay, have a great night and get ready for a great back and bicep workout tomorrow.

Round 11 - Day 5

Are you ready to rock your back and biceps? I bet you are but before you do make certain that your day starts with three very important things: Drink 10-12 ounces of water the minute you get up, eat a well rounded breakfast of good quality food, and fill that head with positive thoughts. If you do those three things, you'll get a great head start to your day. Oh yeah; feed, water, and love those pets too.

That One Thing

Think about one part of your career you have improved by doing 12 Rounds, write it down here, and share it with someone today.

One thing I have improved with my career by doing 12 Rounds is…

____

Seeing I to Eye

Right before your workout today, take 5-6 minutes visualizing yourself doing a few of your exercises with perfect form, being strong, having very high energy, and smiling as you do it. Remember to add one of your favorite songs.

Your Workout – See your workout log for today's workout.

And the Heart Says…

Tonight after dinner and when you have been relaxing for about an hour, take and record a heart rate. Start looking back at your earlier rounds and see what's changed with your heart rates.

Evening resting HR ______ Time taken ______

Cleaning Your Plate

Is it okay to drink caffeine and if so, how much is safe?

I think drinking caffeine is fine as long as it is within safe limits and there is no interaction with medications you may be taking. The Mayo Clinic says up to 400 milligrams (mg) of caffeine a day appears to be safe for most healthy adults. That's roughly the amount of caffeine in four cups of brewed coffee, 10 cans of cola or two "energy shot" drinks.

Although caffeine use may be safe for adults, it's not a good idea for children. And adolescents should limit themselves to no more than 100 mg of caffeine a day.

Many pre-workout drinks have a ton of caffeine in them so be sure to check these amounts to see if they exceed the 400mg level before you get all hyped up.

You Ate What???

Remember to order your food with sauce on the side, steamed, baked or grilled, and ask for no oil or butter in the cooking process. To reduce calories, especially carbs and fat calories, avoid eating chips and bread before your dinner at restaurants; this is where many people get way off track.

Food Journal

Time of meal 1 - _________

Food eaten- ____

Drink - ________________________

Carbohydrates		**Protein**		**Fat**	
Total crab grams -		Total protein grams -		Total fat grams -	
Total fiber grams -		Total protein calories -		Total fat calories	
Total sugar grams -				Total saturated	
Total complex grams -				Total unsaturated -	
Total carb calories -					
Percentage of meal -	%	Percentage of meal -	%	Percentage of meal -	%

Total calories of meal - **cal**
Total ounces of water with meal - **ounces**
Total sodium of meal - **mgs**

Time of meal 2 - _________

Food eaten- ____

Drink - ________________________

Carbohydrates		**Protein**		**Fat**	
Total crab grams -		Total protein grams -		Total fat grams -	
Total fiber grams -		Total protein calories -		Total fat calories	
Total sugar grams -				Total saturated	
Total complex grams -				Total unsaturated -	
Total carb calories -					
Percentage of meal -	%	Percentage of meal -	%	Percentage of meal -	%

Total calories of meal - **cal**
Total ounces of water with meal - **ounces**
Total sodium of meal - **mgs**

Time of meal 3 (Lunch) - _________

Food eaten- ____

Drink - ________________________

Carbohydrates		**Protein**		**Fat**	
Total crab grams -		Total protein grams -		Total fat grams -	
Total fiber grams -		Total protein calories -		Total fat calories	
Total sugar grams -				Total saturated	
Total complex grams -				Total unsaturated -	
Total carb calories -					
Percentage of meal -	%	Percentage of meal -	%	Percentage of meal -	%

Total calories of meal - **cal**
Total ounces of water with meal - **ounces**
Total sodium of meal - **mgs**

Time of meal 4 - _________

Food eaten- ____

Drink - ________________________

Carbohydrates		**Protein**		**Fat**	
Total crab grams -		Total protein grams -		Total fat grams -	
Total fiber grams -		Total protein calories -		Total fat calories	
Total sugar grams -				Total saturated	
Total complex grams -				Total unsaturated -	
Total carb calories -					
Percentage of meal -	%	Percentage of meal -	%	Percentage of meal -	%

Total calories of meal - **cal**
Total ounces of water with meal - **ounces**
Total sodium of meal - **mgs**

Time of meal 5 - _________

Food eaten- ____

Drink - ________________________

Carbohydrates		**Protein**		**Fat**	
Total crab grams -		Total protein grams -		Total fat grams -	
Total fiber grams -		Total protein calories -		Total fat calories	
Total sugar grams -				Total saturated	
Total complex grams -				Total unsaturated -	
Total carb calories -					
Percentage of meal -	%	Percentage of meal -	%	Percentage of meal -	%

Total calories of meal - **cal**
Total ounces of water with meal - **ounces**
Total sodium of meal - **mgs**

Total ounces of water with meals - **ounces**
Total ounces of water during workout - **ounces**
Total ounces of water outside meals - **ounces**
Total ounces of water today - **ounces**
Total sodium today - **mgs**

Here's an idea for you; find someone to start journaling their food with you and pick one day a week to get together and go over each other's journal. It adds accountability and it's a great way to get new ideas for healthy recipes. You can send those to me too.

Round 11 - Day 6

Today's another core and cardio day and this workout is going to challenge you. Get that food in you, get your mind right, and let's go make this the best core and cardio workout yet!

Which Way You Headed?

Write your three long term goals about your career and while you're at it, write down two things you can do over the next two weeks to reach each goal.

Goal 1 - ______________________________

The first thing I can do over the next two weeks to reach this goal is…

____

The second thing I can do over the next two weeks to reach this goal is…

____

Goal 2 - ______________________________

The first thing I can do over the next two weeks to reach this goal is…

____

The second thing I can do over the next two weeks to reach this goal is…

____

Goal 3 - ______________________________

The first thing I can do over the next two weeks to reach this goal is…

____

The second thing I can do over the next two weeks to reach this goal is…

____

Upper Management

One way stress gets the best of us is when we carry it from one place to the next like from work to home. And when you get home, there may just be more stress waiting for you which doesn't leave much room in that head of yours. Start making it a point to take 5-10 minutes on your way home and rid your mind of your days work. I know this can be very challenging but give it your best shot. You can put on some great music, think about something positive, and train your brain to leave work at work.

Seeing I to Eye

How fast can you run? As fast as you want! Take 5-6 minutes today in that quiet place and once your set in and there are no distractions, visualize yourself running at a high rate of speed. You can run through the woods, through a city, beside a river, over the mountains, down the beach, or anywhere else you want. You can even run barefooted if you want and feel the ground beneath your feet. Go ahead; run like the roadrunner.

Your Workout – See your workout log for today's workout.

And the Heart Says…

At some point this evening when you are relaxed, take another heart rate and record it here.

Post workout evening HR ______ Time taken __________

Cleaning Your Plate

So, which one is it? Are egg yolks bad or good for us?

Not only are eggs a fantastic source of lean protein and heart-healthy omega-3 fatty acids, but they contain some pretty important nutrients. And just like any food, you have to be careful of how much you eat.

One large egg has roughly 186 milligrams of cholesterol — all of which is found in the egg's yolk. Since dietary cholesterol was once thought to be the major cause of unhealthy blood cholesterol, egg yolks have been labeled as "bad" so many people avoided the yolk and stuck to eating only the egg white. As long as you haven't been advised otherwise by your doctor, you can enjoy the many nutritional benefits of a whole egg. The egg yolk is also a great source of vitamin D.

Many nutrition experts say that most of us can get by with eating one yolk a day and I agree; as long as a person does not have an existing cholesterol problem. As always, check with your doctor; I'm sure they are going to tell you the same thing.

You Ate What???

If your protein ratio is a little low, try using a protein drink during your two "in between meals" (meals, 2 and 4) to increase your percentage of protein you're consuming. Make sure you're keeping up with your ratios so you can make your diet just right.

Food Journal

Time of meal 1 - _________

Food eaten- ____

Drink - ________________________

Carbohydrates	**Protein**	**Fat**
Total crab grams -	Total protein grams -	Total fat grams -
Total fiber grams -	Total protein calories -	Total fat calories
Total sugar grams -		Total saturated
Total complex grams -		Total unsaturated -
Total carb calories -		
Percentage of meal - %	Percentage of meal - %	Percentage of meal - %

Total calories of meal - cal
Total ounces of water with meal - ounces
Total sodium of meal - mgs

Time of meal 2 - _________

Food eaten- ____

Drink - ________________________

Carbohydrates		**Protein**		**Fat**	
Total crab grams -		Total protein grams -		Total fat grams -	
Total fiber grams -		Total protein calories -		Total fat calories	
Total sugar grams -				Total saturated	
Total complex grams -				Total unsaturated -	
Total carb calories -					
Percentage of meal -	%	Percentage of meal -	%	Percentage of meal -	%

Total calories of meal - **cal**
Total ounces of water with meal - **ounces**
Total sodium of meal - **mgs**

Time of meal 3 (Lunch) - _________

Food eaten- ____

Drink - ________________________

Carbohydrates		**Protein**		**Fat**	
Total crab grams -		Total protein grams -		Total fat grams -	
Total fiber grams -		Total protein calories -		Total fat calories	
Total sugar grams -				Total saturated	
Total complex grams -				Total unsaturated -	
Total carb calories -					
Percentage of meal -	%	Percentage of meal -	%	Percentage of meal -	%

Total calories of meal - **cal**
Total ounces of water with meal - **ounces**
Total sodium of meal - **mgs**

Time of meal 4 - _________

Food eaten- ____

Drink - ________________________

Carbohydrates		**Protein**		**Fat**	
Total crab grams -		Total protein grams -		Total fat grams -	
Total fiber grams -		Total protein calories -		Total fat calories	
Total sugar grams -				Total saturated	
Total complex grams -				Total unsaturated -	
Total carb calories -					
Percentage of meal -	%	Percentage of meal -	%	Percentage of meal -	%

Total calories of meal - **cal**
Total ounces of water with meal - **ounces**
Total sodium of meal - **mgs**

Time of meal 5 - _________

Food eaten- ____

Drink - ________________________

Carbohydrates		**Protein**		**Fat**	
Total crab grams -		Total protein grams -		Total fat grams -	
Total fiber grams -		Total protein calories -		Total fat calories	
Total sugar grams -				Total saturated	
Total complex grams -				Total unsaturated -	
Total carb calories -					
Percentage of meal -	%	Percentage of meal -	%	Percentage of meal -	%

Total calories of meal - **cal**
Total ounces of water with meal - **ounces**
Total sodium of meal - **mgs**

Total ounces of water with meals - **ounces**
Total ounces of water during workout - **ounces**
Total ounces of water outside meals - **ounces**
Total ounces of water today - **ounces**
Total sodium today - **mgs**

It's been a great day for you and now it's time to relax, have some fun, and enjoy your success with 12 Rounds. Speaking of 12 Rounds, we start Round 12 in two days; are you ready to see what I've got in store you? It'll be here before you know it so hold tight and as always, keep positive thoughts in your head, get some good rest, and I'll see you tomorrow for Day 7.

Round 11- Day 7

This is another day off for you and although you already know this, you don't have to keep track of anything today. But just in case you want to, it's here for you to do so. I'll see you tomorrow for Round 12!

I took this heart rate when I was… ____

Day 7 HR ______ **Time taken** _______

Food Journal

Time of meal 1 - _________

Food eaten- ____

Drink - ________________________

Carbohydrates	**Protein**	**Fat**
Total crab grams -	Total protein grams -	Total fat grams -
Total fiber grams -	Total protein calories -	Total fat calories
Total sugar grams -		Total saturated
Total complex grams -		Total unsaturated -
Total carb calories -		
Percentage of meal - %	Percentage of meal - %	Percentage of meal - %

Total calories of meal - cal
Total ounces of water with meal - ounces
Total sodium of meal - mgs

Time of meal 2 - _________

Food eaten- ____

Drink - ________________________

Carbohydrates	**Protein**	**Fat**
Total crab grams -	Total protein grams -	Total fat grams -
Total fiber grams -	Total protein calories -	Total fat calories
Total sugar grams -		Total saturated
Total complex grams -		Total unsaturated -
Total carb calories -		
Percentage of meal - %	Percentage of meal - %	Percentage of meal - %

Total calories of meal - cal
Total ounces of water with meal - ounces
Total sodium of meal - mgs

Time of meal 3 (Lunch) - _________

Food eaten- ____

Drink - ________________________

Carbohydrates	**Protein**	**Fat**
Total crab grams -	Total protein grams -	Total fat grams -
Total fiber grams -	Total protein calories -	Total fat calories
Total sugar grams -		Total saturated
Total complex grams -		Total unsaturated -
Total carb calories -		
Percentage of meal - %	Percentage of meal - %	Percentage of meal - %

Total calories of meal - cal
Total ounces of water with meal - ounces
Total sodium of meal - mgs

Time of meal 4 - ________

Food eaten- ____

Drink - ________________________

Carbohydrates		**Protein**		**Fat**	
Total crab grams -		Total protein grams -		Total fat grams -	
Total fiber grams -		Total protein calories -		Total fat calories	
Total sugar grams -				Total saturated	
Total complex grams -				Total unsaturated -	
Total carb calories -					
Percentage of meal -	%	Percentage of meal -	%	Percentage of meal -	%

Total calories of meal - **cal**
Total ounces of water with meal - **ounces**
Total sodium of meal - **mgs**

Time of meal 5 - ________

Food eaten- ____

Drink - ________________________

Carbohydrates		**Protein**		**Fat**	
Total crab grams -		Total protein grams -		Total fat grams -	
Total fiber grams -		Total protein calories -		Total fat calories	
Total sugar grams -				Total saturated	
Total complex grams -				Total unsaturated -	
Total carb calories -					
Percentage of meal -	%	Percentage of meal -	%	Percentage of meal -	%

Total calories of meal - **cal**
Total ounces of water with meal - **ounces**
Total sodium of meal - **mgs**

Total ounces of water with meals - **ounces**
Total ounces of water during workout - **ounces**
Total ounces of water outside meals - **ounces**
Total ounces of water today - **ounces**
Total sodium today - **mgs**

Round 12 – Fight To WIN!

Day 1

There's one certain thing I know about life; we will all have our battles to fight. And no matter what your battles are, if you fight with everything you have, regardless of the outcome, you'll always come out a winner. With this 12th round, I want you to give me everything you've got and pour your heart into the next seven days. I'm going to be right there with you, and that my friend is an unbeatable team. Let's turn it up!

"Fighting is a big part of life; you're either fighting for things you want, or you're fighting to stay away from things you don't want. Either way, if you want to get to where you really want to go in life, fighting is how you'll get there." ***Bobby Whisnand***

It Happened Just Like This!

In the introduction of 12 Rounds, I told you about the gym I built in my garage, but little did I know, it was the start of building something much bigger. Many people do not know this about me but I struggled with self image for several years of my younger life. Through high school, college, and few years after, I was extremely embarrassed by how I looked physically and I wanted nothing more than to be satisfied with my body. I avoided situations where I would have to wear shorts or take my shirt off, I always walked behind people so not to be noticed, and I tried to workout at times when nobody else would be there. If I went somewhere and happened to see myself in a mirror or reflection from a window, I would immediately leave and feel dejected about how I looked. Some days were better than others but most of the time, it was a tough go. But you know what...I'm glad I went through those struggles and the countless emotional days because little did I know, I was building something that was going to define every single thing about me today; being tough, fighting the fight, and never ever giving up.

No matter how hard things may get in your life, no matter how helpless you may feel at times, and no matter how defeated you may feel, stand back up, grit your teeth, and fight like the champion you are!

That One Thing

On the very first day of this program you wrote down one thing you wanted to achieve the most. Look back to that first day and read what you wrote. Write that one thing down again here and below it, write whether or not you achieved what you wanted the most.

The one thing I wanted to achieve the most with 12 Rounds is...

____

Seeing I to Eye

Are you a sports fan? I hope you are, but even if you're not, here's the scenario I want you to visualize. You're the coach of a football team, it's half time of the championship game, and you're team is down by three touchdowns. Put yourself in front of that team and visualize giving them the speech that will fire them up to go back out there and fight like crazy to take the game back. You're the coach; now lead your team to victory.

Your Workout – See your workout log for today's workout.

And the Heart Says…

After you take this heart rate, take a look back at your heart rates during the first two rounds and see what the difference is.

Pre Sleep HR - ______ Time taken ________

Cleaning Your Plate

Do you know what your blood and cholesterol numbers should be?

This may seem out of place to you, but these are the two biggest reasons to clean up your eating. By the way; when was the last time you had these numbers checked? If it's been a while, schedule a doctor's visit to get them checked. Do we have a deal? Good!

Here are some numbers on healthy and unhealthy blood pressure readings. The top number is the systolic and the bottom number is the diastolic.

- Under 120/80 = normal
- 120-139/80-89 = Pre hypertension
- 140-159/90-99 = Stage 1 hypertension
- 160/100 – Stage 2 hypertension

Here are the ranges for your total cholesterol

- Less than 200mg/dl = desirable
- 200-239 mg/dl = borderline high risk
- 240 and over = high risk

You Ate What???

Remember, changing the way you eat for the better takes time and isn't going to happen overnight so keep at it; it will all come together.

Food Journal

Time of meal 1 - _________

Food eaten- ____

Drink - ________________________

Carbohydrates		**Protein**		**Fat**	
Total crab grams -		Total protein grams -		Total fat grams -	
Total fiber grams -		Total protein calories -		Total fat calories	
Total sugar grams -				Total saturated	
Total complex grams -				Total unsaturated -	
Total carb calories -					
Percentage of meal -	%	Percentage of meal -	%	Percentage of meal -	%

Total calories of meal - **cal**
Total ounces of water with meal - **ounces**
Total sodium of meal - **mgs**

Time of meal 2 - ________

Food eaten- ____

Drink - ________________________

Carbohydrates		**Protein**		**Fat**	
Total carb grams -		Total protein grams -		Total fat grams -	
Total fiber grams -		Total protein calories -		Total fat calories	
Total sugar grams -				Total saturated	
Total complex grams -				Total unsaturated -	
Total carb calories -					
Percentage of meal -	%	Percentage of meal -	%	Percentage of meal -	%

Total calories of meal - **cal**
Total ounces of water with meal - **ounces**
Total sodium of meal - **mgs**

Time of meal 3 (Lunch) - ________

Food eaten- ____

Drink - ________________________

Carbohydrates		**Protein**		**Fat**	
Total carb grams -		Total protein grams -		Total fat grams -	
Total fiber grams -		Total protein calories -		Total fat calories	
Total sugar grams -				Total saturated	
Total complex grams -				Total unsaturated -	
Total carb calories -					
Percentage of meal -	%	Percentage of meal -	%	Percentage of meal -	%

Total calories of meal - **cal**
Total ounces of water with meal - **ounces**
Total sodium of meal - **mgs**

Time of meal 4 - _________

Food eaten- ____

Drink - ________________________

Carbohydrates		**Protein**		**Fat**	
Total carb grams -		Total protein grams -		Total fat grams -	
Total fiber grams -		Total protein calories -		Total fat calories	
Total sugar grams -				Total saturated	
Total complex grams -				Total unsaturated -	
Total carb calories -					
Percentage of meal -	%	Percentage of meal -	%	Percentage of meal -	%

Total calories of meal - **cal**
Total ounces of water with meal - **ounces**
Total sodium of meal - **mgs**

Time of meal 5 - _________

Food eaten- ____

Drink - ________________________

Carbohydrates		**Protein**		**Fat**	
Total carb grams -		Total protein grams -		Total fat grams -	
Total fiber grams -		Total protein calories -		Total fat calories	
Total sugar grams -				Total saturated	
Total complex grams -				Total unsaturated -	
Total carb calories -					
Percentage of meal -	%	Percentage of meal -	%	Percentage of meal -	%

Total calories of meal - **cal**
Total ounces of water with meal - **ounces**
Total sodium of meal - **mgs**

Total ounces of water with meals - **ounces**
Total ounces of water during workout - **ounces**
Total ounces of water outside meals - **ounces**
Total ounces of water today - **ounces**
Total sodium today - **mgs**

Now that's the way to start Round 12; way to go! Now let's set our sights on Day 2; are you with me?

Round 12 - Day 2

How's that six pack coming along? Is it there and you just can't see it yet, or is it peaking through? Either way, keep at it because they will show up one day soon. Let's go do this Day 2

Which Way You Headed?

Write your three long term goals about something other than your fitness and underneath the ones you haven't reached yet, write down something you can do to reach it over the next 6 days.

Goal 1 - ____

To reach this goal in the next 6 days, I need to…

____

Goal 2 - ____

To reach this goal in the next 6 days, I need to…

____

Goal 3 - ____

To reach this goal in the next 6 days, I need to…

____

Seeing I to Eye

Here's a good one for you: You're hired to speak to an elementary school; what's your topic? Once you have your topic write it down here and take 5-6 minutes visualizing yourself giving those kids your speech.

My speech to an elementary school would be about …

____

Upper Management

Throughout this program you've learned some things to help manage your stress. What do you feel were a few of the most effective things you used over these 12 Rounds that truly reduced your stress?

The things I used with 12 Rounds that helped me the most to manage my stress were…

____

____

____

Your Workout – See your workout log for today's workout.

Cleaning Your Plate

What are electrolytes and how do I get them?

There are several common electrolytes found in the body, each serving a specific and important role, but most are in some part responsible for maintaining the balance of fluids between the intracellular (inside the cell) and extracellular (outside the cell) environments. This balance is critically important for things like hydration, nerve impulses, muscle function, and pH level.

Here is a list of electrolytes

- Sodium, Chloride, Potassium, Magnesium, Calcium, Phosphate, Bicarbonate

Okay, so what's the best way to get these in your body? You may think of getting a re-surge in electrolytes from sports drinks, but the best and most natural way of replenishing electrolytes is from food. In fact, sugary sports drinks only provide a quick burst of minerals, and they deplete the body over time. Foods that contain a good amount of electrolytes are fruits and vegetables, nuts and seeds, beans, bananas, and dark leafy greens.

You Ate What???

As you can see from above, fruits and vegetables play a very important role in your nutrition and that's exactly why you should shoot for making half your plate fruits and non starchy vegetables. Start taking a close look at how many starchy carbs you're eating versus non starchy carbs. You do need some of these starchy carbs but if you eat too many, it can cause you to gain unwanted weight. If gaining weight is your goal, increase the amount of starchy carbs in your diet. For a refresher on starchy carbs, look back at Day 6 of Round 6.

Food Journal

Time of meal 1 - ________

Food eaten- ____

Drink - ________________________

Carbohydrates		**Protein**		**Fat**	
Total crab grams -		Total protein grams -		Total fat grams -	
Total fiber grams -		Total protein calories -		Total fat calories	
Total sugar grams -				Total saturated	
Total complex grams -				Total unsaturated -	
Total carb calories -					
Percentage of meal -	%	Percentage of meal -	%	Percentage of meal -	%

Total calories of meal - **cal**
Total ounces of water with meal - **ounces**
Total sodium of meal - **mgs**

Time of meal 2 - ________

Food eaten- ____

Drink - ________________________

Carbohydrates		Protein		Fat	
Total carb grams -		Total protein grams -		Total fat grams -	
Total fiber grams -		Total protein calories -		Total fat calories	
Total sugar grams -				Total saturated	
Total complex grams -				Total unsaturated -	
Total carb calories -					
Percentage of meal -	%	Percentage of meal -	%	Percentage of meal -	%

Total calories of meal - **cal**
Total ounces of water with meal - **ounces**
Total sodium of meal - **mgs**

Time of meal 3 (Lunch) - ________

Food eaten- ____

Drink - ________________________

Carbohydrates		Protein		Fat	
Total carb grams -		Total protein grams -		Total fat grams -	
Total fiber grams -		Total protein calories -		Total fat calories	
Total sugar grams -				Total saturated	
Total complex grams -				Total unsaturated -	
Total carb calories -					
Percentage of meal -	%	Percentage of meal -	%	Percentage of meal -	%

Total calories of meal - **cal**
Total ounces of water with meal - **ounces**
Total sodium of meal - **mgs**

Time of meal 4 - ________

Food eaten- ____

Drink - ________________________

Carbohydrates		Protein		Fat	
Total carb grams -		Total protein grams -		Total fat grams -	
Total fiber grams -		Total protein calories -		Total fat calories	
Total sugar grams -				Total saturated	
Total complex grams -				Total unsaturated -	
Total carb calories -					
Percentage of meal -	%	Percentage of meal -	%	Percentage of meal -	%

Total calories of meal - **cal**
Total ounces of water with meal - **ounces**
Total sodium of meal - **mgs**

Time of meal 5 - ________

Food eaten- ____

Drink - ________________________

Carbohydrates		**Protein**		**Fat**	
Total carb grams -		Total protein grams -		Total fat grams -	
Total fiber grams -		Total protein calories -		Total fat calories	
Total sugar grams -				Total saturated	
Total complex grams -				Total unsaturated -	
Total carb calories -					
Percentage of meal -	%	Percentage of meal -	%	Percentage of meal -	%

Total calories of meal - cal
Total ounces of water with meal - ounces
Total sodium of meal - mgs

Total ounces of water with meals - ounces
Total ounces of water during workout - ounces
Total ounces of water outside meals - ounces
Total ounces of water today - ounces
Total sodium today - mgs

And The Heart Says…

At some point in the middle of your day, take a heart rate and record it here.

Afternoon HR-________ Time taken - _______

Nutrition is a very big part of making healthier choices and I hope you have learned some very valuable things with 12 Rounds to help you eat better. Speaking of eating, isn't it time for you to eat dinner? Make sure you keep those complex carbs low and replace them with protein and green vegetables for your dinner if you're trying to lose weight. If you're trying to gain weight, throw some clean complex carbs in there like brown rice, quinoa, or a sweet potato. But either way, don't forget to write everything down. I'll see you tomorrow for the almighty leg day!

Round 12 – Day 3

There you arc; How was that sleep? If you're having trouble getting to sleep or staying asleep, try using your visualization skills to put your mind at ease before you go to sleep. But for now, let's go have your best leg day yet. It's a long one so be ready.

That One Thing

On Day 3, you wrote whether or not you achieved what you wanted the most with this program. Today, write another thing you would like to achieve by doing 12 Rounds again.

For my next 12 Rounds, what I want to achieve the most is…

____

Seeing I to Eye

A few rounds back, I asked you to visualize being a hero by saving someone from a dangerous situation, helping them through a difficult time, scoring the winning run, or any other heroic action. Go ahead and do it again today and this time, really bring the fireworks.

Your Workout – See your workout log for today's workout.

And the Heart Says…

While you're at work today and sitting at your desk, take a heart rate and write it down here. Make sure you've been sitting for at least 5 minutes before you take it. Also, take a look back at your first few rounds and see if there is a difference in your heart rates.

Resting HR - ______ Time Taken - ________

Cleaning Your Plate

What exactly is a sugar alcohol and is it bad for me?

Sugar alcohols are one type of reduced-calorie sweetener. You can find them in ice creams, cookies, puddings, candies and chewing gum that are labeled as "sugar-free" or "no sugar added." Sugar alcohols provide fewer calories than sugar and have less of an effect on blood glucose than other carbohydrates.

Examples of sugar alcohol are:

Erythritol

Glycerol (also known as glycerin or glycerine)

- hydrogenated starch hydrolysates, isomalt, lactitol, maltitol, mannitol, sorbitol, xylitol

Even though they are called sugar alcohols, they do not contain alcohol.

When you're considering foods with low- or reduced-calorie sweeteners, always check the nutrition facts on the label. Many of the food products containing these types of sweeteners still have a significant amount of carbohydrate, calories, and fat so never consider them a "free food" without checking the label. By comparing the calories in the sugar-free version to the regular version, you'll see whether you're really getting fewer calories.

You Ate What???
If you know someone who is struggling with their eating, show them a few of your food journals from Round 1 and then one from the last few rounds. This way they will know that you can start with a minimal amount of journaling until you get the habit down.

Food Journal

Time of meal 1 - _________

Food eaten- ____

Drink - ________________________

Carbohydrates		**Protein**		**Fat**	
Total crab grams -		Total protein grams -		Total fat grams -	
Total fiber grams -		Total protein calories -		Total fat calories	
Total sugar grams -				Total saturated	
Total complex grams -				Total unsaturated -	
Total carb calories -					
Percentage of meal -	%	Percentage of meal -	%	Percentage of meal -	%

Total calories of meal - **cal**
Total ounces of water with meal - **ounces**
Total sodium of meal - **mgs**

Time of meal 2 - _________

Food eaten- ____

Drink - ________________________

Carbohydrates		**Protein**		**Fat**	
Total carb grams -		Total protein grams -		Total fat grams -	
Total fiber grams -		Total protein calories -		Total fat calories	
Total sugar grams -				Total saturated	
Total complex grams -				Total unsaturated -	
Total carb calories -					
Percentage of meal -	%	Percentage of meal -	%	Percentage of meal -	%

Total calories of meal - **cal**
Total ounces of water with meal - **ounces**
Total sodium of meal - **mgs**

Time of meal 3 (Lunch) - _________

Food eaten- ____

Drink - ________________________

Carbohydrates		**Protein**		**Fat**	
Total carb grams -		Total protein grams -		Total fat grams -	
Total fiber grams -		Total protein calories -		Total fat calories	
Total sugar grams -				Total saturated	
Total complex grams -				Total unsaturated -	
Total carb calories -					
Percentage of meal -	%	Percentage of meal -	%	Percentage of meal -	%

Total calories of meal - **cal**
Total ounces of water with meal - **ounces**
Total sodium of meal - **mgs**

Time of meal 4 - _________

Food eaten- ____

Drink - ________________________

Carbohydrates		**Protein**		**Fat**	
Total carb grams -		Total protein grams -		Total fat grams -	
Total fiber grams -		Total protein calories -		Total fat calories	
Total sugar grams -				Total saturated	
Total complex grams -				Total unsaturated -	
Total carb calories -					
Percentage of meal -	%	Percentage of meal -	%	Percentage of meal -	%

Total calories of meal - **cal**
Total ounces of water with meal - **ounces**
Total sodium of meal - **mgs**

Time of meal 5 - _________

Food eaten- ____

Drink - ________________________

Carbohydrates		**Protein**		**Fat**	
Total carb grams -		Total protein grams -		Total fat grams -	
Total fiber grams -		Total protein calories -		Total fat calories	
Total sugar grams -				Total saturated	
Total complex grams -				Total unsaturated -	
Total carb calories -					
Percentage of meal -	%	Percentage of meal -	%	Percentage of meal -	%

Total calories of meal - **cal**
Total ounces of water with meal - **ounces**
Total sodium of meal - **mgs**

Total ounces of water with meals - **ounces**
Total ounces of water during workout - **ounces**
Total ounces of water outside meals - **ounces**
Total ounces of water today - **ounces**
Total sodium today - **mgs**

Those unilateral leg days are really something aren't they? By the end of that workout, you're ready for some good food and some good sleep; just don't forget to clear you're head while you're at it. I'll see you tomorrow Champ!

Round 12 - Day 4

Here we go; another day to live life, be happy, and have some fun. Let's make it a great one!

"Living life can be a real fight sometimes, but I'll choose the fight every single time. It's when you choose not to fight that living escapes you." ***Bobby Whisnand***

It Happened Just Like This!

This is my last story for you, and I saved the best for last. About a year ago, I started working with a new client who had countless health issues. Her name was Wanda, and she was a cancer survivor. She had severe COPD. Both hips and one knee had been replaced. She had a rod in each leg. She had severe scoliosis, and arthritis from head to toe. By the way; she was 87 years old. For the first two weeks she could only exercise in a seated position for about 4-5 minutes, but after a month, she was able to stand up and exercise for 15-20 minutes. After another month, she was not only exercising for 30-45 minutes at a time, she was doing kick boxing and other cardio combinations like a champ. She was doing so well that her cardiologist told her he didn't need to see her for a whole year; that's a big change from going once a month.

After about a year of working with Wanda, she was diagnosed with Stage IV lymphoma for the second time, but it didn't slow her down much. The day she told me, she looked at me and said, "Bobby, we're going to fight like the dickens, and we're not going to miss one workout; do you hear me?" We didn't miss one workout over the next two months and we did our last workout five days before she passed. Every single time Wanda and I worked out, she would tell me how much I did for her but it was really the other way around. She showed me what toughness was all about, how to keep fighting when life turns you upside down, and the most important thing of all: As long as you keep fighting, you can't lose.

Which Way You Headed?

Write your three long term goals about your fitness and underneath the ones you haven't reached yet, write down something you can do to reach it over the next 4 days.

Goal 1 - ____

To reach this goal in the next 4 days, I need to…

____

Goal 2 - ____

To reach this goal in the next 4 days, I need to…

____

Goal 3 - ____

To reach this goal in the next 4 days, I need to…

____

Seeing I to Eye

Get to that quiet place and visualize the following scenario: You're in a race in a track meet and there are two people in front of you. You're coming around the last turn with nothing but a straight away in front of you. Visualize you passing both of the other runners and as you pass them, see their numbers on the back of their shirts, and then run through the white tape at the finish line with the crowd cheering very loudly. Go do it and see yourself winning!

Upper Management

During Round 2, you wrote a list of things you need to get done. Write that original list here again, mark through the things you got done, and circle the things you still need to do; if there are any. If there are few things left, do your best to mark them off over the next four days.

These are the things I need to get done to lighten my load:

1. ______________________________	7. ______________________________
2. ______________________________	8. ______________________________
3. ______________________________	9. ______________________________
4. ______________________________	10. ______________________________
5. ______________________________	11. ______________________________
6. ______________________________	12. ______________________________

No Workout Today!

And the Heart Says…

Take at least one heart rate today whenever you want. Just make sure you write down when and under what circumstances you took it.

Today I took my heart rate when I was… ____________________________________

Day 4 HR - ______ Time taken - ________

Cleaning Your Plate

Are sweet potatoes healthier than white potatoes?

Both types of potatoes pack a powerful nutritional punch but sweet potatoes provides 400% of your daily requirement of vitamin A. They also have more vitamin C, have fewer calories, more fiber, and fewer total carbs than white potatoes. Both types of potatoes are good for you, but just like with any carbohydrate loaded food, you have to be careful of how much you eat and when you eat them.

You Ate What???

Keep up the good work on your food journal and when you get some time, start taking a look back at some of your food journals from the earlier rounds and see where you're improving.

Food Journal

Time of meal 1 - _________

Food eaten- ____

Drink - ________________________

Carbohydrates		**Protein**		**Fat**	
Total crab grams -		Total protein grams -		Total fat grams -	
Total fiber grams -		Total protein calories -		Total fat calories	
Total sugar grams -				Total saturated	
Total complex grams -				Total unsaturated -	
Total carb calories -					
Percentage of meal -	%	Percentage of meal -	%	Percentage of meal -	%

Total calories of meal - **cal**
Total ounces of water with meal - **ounces**
Total sodium of meal - **mgs**

Time of meal 2 - _________

Food eaten- ____

Drink - ________________________

Carbohydrates		**Protein**		**Fat**	
Total crab grams -		Total protein grams -		Total fat grams -	
Total fiber grams -		Total protein calories -		Total fat calories	
Total sugar grams -				Total saturated	
Total complex grams -				Total unsaturated -	
Total carb calories -					
Percentage of meal -	%	Percentage of meal -	%	Percentage of meal -	%

Total calories of meal - **cal**
Total ounces of water with meal - **ounces**
Total sodium of meal - **mgs**

Time of meal 3 (Lunch) - _________

Food eaten- ____

Drink - ________________________

Carbohydrates		**Protein**		**Fat**	
Total crab grams -		Total protein grams -		Total fat grams -	
Total fiber grams -		Total protein calories -		Total fat calories	
Total sugar grams -				Total saturated	
Total complex grams -				Total unsaturated -	
Total carb calories -					
Percentage of meal -	%	Percentage of meal -	%	Percentage of meal -	%

Total calories of meal - **cal**
Total ounces of water with meal - **ounces**
Total sodium of meal - **mgs**

Time of meal 4 - _________

Food eaten- ____

Drink - ________________________

Carbohydrates		**Protein**		**Fat**	
Total crab grams -		Total protein grams -		Total fat grams -	
Total fiber grams -		Total protein calories -		Total fat calories	
Total sugar grams -				Total saturated	
Total complex grams -				Total unsaturated -	
Total carb calories -					
Percentage of meal -	%	Percentage of meal -	%	Percentage of meal -	%

Total calories of meal - **cal**
Total ounces of water with meal - **ounces**
Total sodium of meal - **mgs**

Time of meal 5 - _________

Food eaten- ____

Drink - ________________________

Carbohydrates		**Protein**		**Fat**	
Total crab grams -		Total protein grams -		Total fat grams -	
Total fiber grams -		Total protein calories -		Total fat calories	
Total sugar grams -				Total saturated	
Total complex grams -				Total unsaturated -	
Total carb calories -					
Percentage of meal -	%	Percentage of meal -	%	Percentage of meal -	%

Total calories of meal - **cal**
Total ounces of water with meal - **ounces**
Total sodium of meal - **mgs**

Total ounces of water with meals - **ounces**
Total ounces of water outside meals - **ounces**
Total ounces of water today - **ounces**
Total sodium today - **mgs**

As you make your way through these next three days, really take some time thinking back to when you first started. This is a good time to start looking back over your workout logs to see where some changes are starting to happen. Believe it or not, your biggest changes are yet to come; you'll see!

Round 12 - Day 5

There's nothing like a great back and bicep workout, especially when you get that good pump and your energy feels like it will never run out. That's how I want all of your workouts to be; great pumps and full of energy. And you know exactly how to make them that way; let's do it again today!

That One Thing

Think of one person you know who you think would like to do 12 Rounds. Once you know who it is, write their name down here.

The one person who I think would love 12 Rounds is…

____

Seeing I to Eye

A company hires you to give a keynote speech to their employees to motivate everyone to do better at work and home. Come up with a title to your high energy presentation and take 5-6 minutes today visualizing giving this presentation to a big audience. Remember; high energy!

Your Workout – See your workout log for today's workout.

And the Heart Says…

Tonight after dinner and when you have been relaxing for about an hour, take and record a heart rate. Start looking back at your earlier rounds and see what's changed with your heart rates.

Evening resting HR ______ Time taken ______

Cleaning Your Plate

What exactly is Cacao chocolate and is it healthy to eat? Is it the same as Cocoa?

Cacao is the purest form of chocolate you can consume, which means it is raw and much less processed than cocoa powder or chocolate bars. Cacao is thought to be the highest source of antioxidants of all foods and the highest source of magnesium of all foods. It has been used throughout many cultures for years for health purposes.

You can use cocoa powder and cacao powder interchangeably in baking recipes, smoothies, oatmeal, cookies, homemade raw treats, or even stir them into your coffee for a homemade mocha. Both cacao and cocoa are highly nutritious for you and are sure to satisfy your chocolate cravings around the clock. If you want more nutrients, I would suggest you choose cacao, but if you want fewer calories and a decent source of antioxidants, then definitely go with cocoa powder.

You Ate What???

Have you greatly reduced the amount of sodium you're consuming since you started journaling your sodium intake? I hope you are because consuming too much sodium (more than 1500mg/day) can lead to one of the silent killers: High blood pressure.

Food Journal

Time of meal 1 - _________

Food eaten- ____

Drink - ________________________

Carbohydrates		**Protein**		**Fat**	
Total crab grams -		Total protein grams -		Total fat grams -	
Total fiber grams -		Total protein calories -		Total fat calories	
Total sugar grams -				Total saturated	
Total complex grams -				Total unsaturated -	
Total carb calories -					
Percentage of meal -	%	Percentage of meal -	%	Percentage of meal -	%
Total calories of meal -		**cal**			
Total ounces of water with meal -		**ounces**			
Total sodium of meal -		**mgs**			

Time of meal 2 - _________

Food eaten- ____

Drink - ________________________

Carbohydrates		**Protein**		**Fat**	
Total crab grams -		Total protein grams -		Total fat grams -	
Total fiber grams -		Total protein calories -		Total fat calories	
Total sugar grams -				Total saturated	
Total complex grams -				Total unsaturated -	
Total carb calories -					
Percentage of meal -	%	Percentage of meal -	%	Percentage of meal -	%
Total calories of meal -		**cal**			
Total ounces of water with meal -		**ounces**			
Total sodium of meal -		**mgs**			

Time of meal 3 (Lunch) - _________

Food eaten- ____

Drink - ________________________

Carbohydrates		**Protein**		**Fat**	
Total carb grams -		Total protein grams -		Total fat grams -	
Total fiber grams -		Total protein calories -		Total fat calories	
Total sugar grams -				Total saturated	
Total complex grams -				Total unsaturated -	
Total carb calories -					
Percentage of meal -	%	Percentage of meal -	%	Percentage of meal -	%
Total calories of meal -		**cal**			
Total ounces of water with meal -		**ounces**			
Total sodium of meal -		**mgs**			

Time of meal 4 - ________

Food eaten- ____

Drink - ________________________

Carbohydrates		**Protein**		**Fat**	
Total carb grams -		Total protein grams -		Total fat grams -	
Total fiber grams -		Total protein calories -		Total fat calories	
Total sugar grams -				Total saturated	
Total complex grams -				Total unsaturated -	
Total carb calories -					
Percentage of meal -	%	Percentage of meal -	%	Percentage of meal -	%

Total calories of meal - **cal**
Total ounces of water with meal - **ounces**
Total sodium of meal - **mgs**

Time of meal 5 - ________

Food eaten- ____

Drink - ________________________

Carbohydrates		**Protein**		**Fat**	
Total carb grams -		Total protein grams -		Total fat grams -	
Total fiber grams -		Total protein calories -		Total fat calories	
Total sugar grams -				Total saturated	
Total complex grams -				Total unsaturated -	
Total carb calories -					
Percentage of meal -	%	Percentage of meal -	%	Percentage of meal -	%

Total calories of meal - **cal**
Total ounces of water with meal - **ounces**
Total sodium of meal - **mgs**

Total ounces of water with meals - **ounces**
Total ounces of water during workout - **ounces**
Total ounces of water outside meals - **ounces**
Total ounces of water today - **ounces**
Total sodium today - **mgs**

Have you noticed a change in your overall outlook on life since you started 12 Rounds? I sure hope you have and even though you may be a very positive person, I hope there were things throughout 12 Rounds that have helped you make it even better. Go get some rest Champ; we've got a big day tomorrow!

Round 12 - Day 6

This is your last core and cardio workout for your very first 12 Rounds. What do you say we knock it out of the park? Well come on then; if you're waiting on me, you're backing up!

Which Way You Headed?

Write your three long term goals about your career and underneath the ones you haven't reached yet, write down something you can do to reach it over the next 2 days.

Goal 1 - ____

To reach this goal in the next 2 days, I need to…

____

Goal 2 - ____

To reach this goal in the next 2 days, I need to…

____

Goal 3 - ____

To reach this goal in the next 2 days, I need to…

____

Upper Management

Go see the people who you counted on for your support through 12 Rounds and thank them for supporting you. Share with them how well you did and better yet, get them to go another 12 Rounds with you. And this time, you can be the coach.

Seeing I to Eye

On Day 1 of 12 Rounds, I asked you to visualize doing something you love to do. Today, I want you to do it again except this time visualize yourself doing it while being in great shape, full of energy, completely content, and smiling from ear to ear. Go ahead; let's see what you've got!

Your Workout – See your workout log for today's workout.

And the Heart Says…

At some point this evening when you are relaxed, take another heart rate and record it here.

Post workout evening HR ______ Time taken __________

Cleaning Your Plate

What's the deal with quinoa? Is it as healthy as everyone says?

Quinoa is a complete protein, wheat free alternative for complex carbohydrates. That's good enough in itself, but there are many other reasons quinoa is so good for you. With twice the protein content of rice or barley, quinoa is also a very good source of calcium, magnesium and manganese. It also possesses good levels of several B vitamins, vitamin E and dietary fiber. Are you convinced yet? Quinoa is among the least allergenic of all the grains, making it a fantastic wheat-free choice. Like buckwheat, quinoa has an excellent amino acid profile, as it contains all nine essential amino acids making it a complete-protein source. Quinoa is therefore an excellent choice for vegans who may struggle to get enough protein in their diets.

Quinoa is also high in anti-inflammatory phytonutrients, which make it potentially beneficial for human health in the prevention and treatment of disease. Quinoa contains small amounts of the heart healthy omega-3 fatty acids and, in comparison to common cereal grasses has a higher content of monounsaturated fat. I eat quinoa on a daily basis and if you haven't ever tried it, be prepared for a very bland tasting food. It goes great with baked fish and pork, but however you eat it, you may need to spice it up a bit.

You Ate What???

One thing you can do to advance your healthy eating is to hire a licensed nutritionist to help you along. If you do so, show them your food journals through 12 Rounds and the progress you've made along the way. If you use someone other than a licensed nutritionist, please use caution because there are a lot of "nutrition experts" out there who are way off the mark.

Food Journal

Time of meal 1 - _________

Food eaten- ____

Drink - ________________________

Carbohydrates		**Protein**		**Fat**	
Total crab grams -		Total protein grams -		Total fat grams -	
Total fiber grams -		Total protein calories -		Total fat calories	
Total sugar grams -				Total saturated	
Total complex grams -				Total unsaturated -	
Total carb calories -					
Percentage of meal -	%	Percentage of meal -	%	Percentage of meal -	%
Total calories of meal -		**cal**			
Total ounces of water with meal -		**ounces**			
Total sodium of meal -		**mgs**			

Time of meal 2 - _________

Food eaten- ____

Drink - ________________________

Carbohydrates		**Protein**		**Fat**	
Total crab grams -		Total protein grams -		Total fat grams -	
Total fiber grams -		Total protein calories -		Total fat calories	
Total sugar grams -				Total saturated	
Total complex grams -				Total unsaturated -	
Total carb calories -					
Percentage of meal -	%	Percentage of meal -	%	Percentage of meal -	%
Total calories of meal -		**cal**			
Total ounces of water with meal -		**ounces**			
Total sodium of meal -		**mgs**			

Time of meal 3 (Lunch) - ________

Food eaten- ____

Drink - ____________________

Carbohydrates		**Protein**		**Fat**	
Total crab grams -		Total protein grams -		Total fat grams -	
Total fiber grams -		Total protein calories -		Total fat calories	
Total sugar grams -				Total saturated	
Total complex grams -				Total unsaturated -	
Total carb calories -					
Percentage of meal -	%	Percentage of meal -	%	Percentage of meal -	%

Total calories of meal - **cal**
Total ounces of water with meal - **ounces**
Total sodium of meal - **mgs**

Time of meal 4 - ________

Food eaten- ____

Drink - ____________________

Carbohydrates		**Protein**		**Fat**	
Total crab grams -		Total protein grams -		Total fat grams -	
Total fiber grams -		Total protein calories -		Total fat calories	
Total sugar grams -				Total saturated	
Total complex grams -				Total unsaturated -	
Total carb calories -					
Percentage of meal -	%	Percentage of meal -	%	Percentage of meal -	%

Total calories of meal - **cal**
Total ounces of water with meal - **ounces**
Total sodium of meal - **mgs**

Time of meal 5 - ________

Food eaten- ____

Drink - ____________________

Carbohydrates		**Protein**		**Fat**	
Total crab grams -		Total protein grams -		Total fat grams -	
Total fiber grams -		Total protein calories -		Total fat calories	
Total sugar grams -				Total saturated	
Total complex grams -				Total unsaturated -	
Total carb calories -					
Percentage of meal -	%	Percentage of meal -	%	Percentage of meal -	%

Total calories of meal - **cal**
Total ounces of water with meal - **ounces**
Total sodium of meal - **mgs**

Total ounces of water with meals - ounces
Total ounces of water during workout - ounces
Total ounces of water outside meals - ounces
Total ounces of water today - ounces
Total sodium today - mgs

And just like that; Day 6 of Round 12 is in the books. How did you do with your core and cardio circuit today? Like I said before, even though you may not be doing a "cardio type activity" you can still be in an aerobic state. That's why I paired your core exercises in a circuit with cardio activity throughout 12 Rounds. Go get some good sleep and I'll see you tomorrow to close out your first 12 Rounds.

Round 12- Day 7

Good morning! How are your abs feeling today? Did you get enough sleep last night? This is your last day with your first 12 Rounds and as usual, you don't have to do anything but enjoy your day. However, I do have a few things I want you to do tomorrow so make sure you take a look. Okay, go make it a great day; you definitely know how to do that by now.

I took this heart rate when I was... ______________________________

Day 7 HR ______ Time taken _______

Food Journal

Time of meal 1 - _________

Food eaten- ______________________________

Drink - ________________

Carbohydrates	**Protein**	**Fat**
Total crab grams -	Total protein grams -	Total fat grams -
Total fiber grams -	Total protein calories -	Total fat calories
Total sugar grams -		Total saturated
Total complex grams -		Total unsaturated -
Total carb calories -		
Percentage of meal - %	Percentage of meal - %	Percentage of meal - %

Total calories of meal - cal
Total ounces of water with meal - ounces
Total sodium of meal - mgs

Time of meal 2 - _________

Food eaten- ______________________________

Drink - ________________

Carbohydrates		**Protein**		**Fat**	
Total crab grams -		Total protein grams -		Total fat grams -	
Total fiber grams -		Total protein calories -		Total fat calories	
Total sugar grams -				Total saturated	
Total complex grams -				Total unsaturated -	
Total carb calories -					
Percentage of meal -	%	Percentage of meal -	%	Percentage of meal -	%

Total calories of meal - **cal**
Total ounces of water with meal - **ounces**
Total sodium of meal - **mgs**

Time of meal 3 (Lunch) - _________

Food eaten- ____

Drink - ________________________

Carbohydrates		**Protein**		**Fat**	
Total crab grams -		Total protein grams -		Total fat grams -	
Total fiber grams -		Total protein calories -		Total fat calories	
Total sugar grams -				Total saturated	
Total complex grams -				Total unsaturated -	
Total carb calories -					
Percentage of meal -	%	Percentage of meal -	%	Percentage of meal -	%

Total calories of meal - **cal**
Total ounces of water with meal - **ounces**
Total sodium of meal - **mgs**

Time of meal 4 - _________

Food eaten- ____

Drink - ________________________

Carbohydrates		**Protein**		**Fat**	
Total crab grams -		Total protein grams -		Total fat grams -	
Total fiber grams -		Total protein calories -		Total fat calories	
Total sugar grams -				Total saturated	
Total complex grams -				Total unsaturated -	
Total carb calories -					
Percentage of meal -	%	Percentage of meal -	%	Percentage of meal -	%

Total calories of meal - **cal**
Total ounces of water with meal - **ounces**
Total sodium of meal - **mgs**

Time of meal 5 - _________

Food eaten- ____

Drink - ________________________

Carbohydrates		**Protein**		**Fat**	
Total crab grams -		Total protein grams -		Total fat grams -	
Total fiber grams -		Total protein calories -		Total fat calories	
Total sugar grams -				Total saturated	
Total complex grams -				Total unsaturated -	
Total carb calories -					
Percentage of meal -	%	Percentage of meal -	%	Percentage of meal -	%

Total calories of meal - **cal**
Total ounces of water with meal - **ounces**
Total sodium of meal - **mgs**

Total ounces of water with meals - **ounces**
Total ounces of water outside meals - **ounces**
Total ounces of water today - **ounces**
Total sodium today - **mgs**

Coming up next, Round 13! Are you ready for it? Actually, there is no Round 13, but there is another amazing 12 Rounds waiting on you. I know you've made some great progress with your first 12 Rounds, but believe it or not, your next 12 Rounds is where you'll make your biggest improvements yet. It's these next 12 Rounds where you'll see greater gains in strength, better eating habits, and a much stronger mind to take you farther in life than you've ever been. But before you get going, there are some things I want you to do to make sure that these next 12 Rounds will be as good as they can be, and I have listed them here:

- ➔ Find someone or multiple people to do the next 12 Rounds with you and help them have the success you've had. You can even get together once a week to support each other.
- ➔ If you haven't reached all of the goals you set during the first 12 Rounds, write those goals down at the beginning and do your best to overcome the reasons these goals weren't met. For the ones you've reached, set new ones and keep moving on.
- ➔ You can use the same visualizations you used the first time around or you can come up with some new ones. Either way, keep seeing I to eye.
- ➔ For your workout journal you can order a brand new complete 12 week journal to use on your next 12 Rounds.
- ➔ You now have a comparison for all 36 workouts you did during 12 Rounds. Use these your next time around and as long as your form is great and you're doing all repetitions by going slow, you can increase the resistance by small increments for each of your next 36 workouts.
- ➔ For your heart rates, you can record them right beside the first ones, or you can use your notebook for these as well.
- ➔ Reward yourself; you did awesome!

Success means different things to many people, but I hope in your eyes and your heart, you feel much more in control of your life, you've found new confidence to do things you never thought you could do, and you feel more alive than you ever have after going through 12 Rounds with me. Oh yea; there's one more thing. I hope one day down the road, you think back to where it all started by a skinny kid who built a little gym out of wood, plumbing pipe, and cable in a hot unventilated garage in Iowa Park, Texas. Where the 3rd hand mismatched concrete weights were piled in the floor, the bars were bent and rusty, where a young man's confidence was found, and the makings of the best fitness program in the world was born.

Here is another body measurement form in case you're tracking these.

End of 12 Rounds Body Measurements

- **Date of measurements** - ____________________
- **Body weight** - _________ lbs
- **Body fat%** - ___________%
- **Shoulders** (measure across mid shoulder line) - _______
- **Chest** (measure across nipple line) - ________
- **Upper arm** (measure across mid bicep) - _______
- **Forearm** (measure across mid forearm between wrist and elbow) - _______
- **Waist** (measure right across belly button) - ________
- **Hips** (measure across mid buttocks) - ________
- **Upper thigh** (measure across mid upper thigh) - ________
- **Lower thigh** (measure across just above knee) - _______
- **Calf (measure across mid calf) - _______**